New Ways of Using Drama and Literature in Language Teaching

Valerie Whiteson, Editor

New Ways in TESOL Series II
Innovative Classroom Techniques
Jack C. Richards, Series Editor

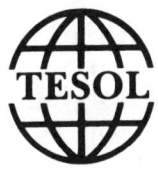

Teachers of English to Speakers of Other Languages, Inc.

Typeset in Garamond Book and Tiffany Demi
by Capitol Communication Systems, Inc., Crofton, Maryland USA
and printed by
Pantagraph Printing, Bloomington, Illinois USA

Teachers of English to Speakers of Other Languages, Inc. (TESOL)
1600 Cameron Street, Suite 300
Alexandria, VA 22314 USA
Tel 703-836-0774 • Fax 703-836-7864

Director of Communications and Marketing: Helen Kornblum
Senior Editor: Marilyn Kupetz
Copy Editor: Ellen Garshick
Editorial Assistant: Cheryl Donnelly
Cover Design and Spot Art: Ann Kammerer

Copyright © 1996 by Teachers of English to Speakers of Other Languages, Inc.

All rights reserved. No part of this publication may be reproduced or transmitted in any form or by any means, electronic or mechanical, including photocopy, or any informational storage or retrieval system, without permission from the publisher.

Every effort has been made to contact the copyright holders for permission to reprint borrowed material. We regret any oversights that may have occurred and will rectify them in future printings of this work.

TESOL thanks Michael Carrier, the staff, and the students at Eurocentres, Alexandria, Virginia, for their participation and assistance.

ISBN 939791-66-8
Library of Congress Catalogue No. 96-061035

To my teachers in the English department at Bar Ilan University, who inspired me to love literature and learning

Contents

Acknowledgments vi
Introduction vii
Users' Guide to Activities ix
Part I: Prose 1
Part II: Poetry 63
Part III: Drama 87
Part IV: A Mixed Bag 129

Acknowledgments

I would like to thank Jack Richards, Series Editor, for the opportunity to edit this volume; Helen Kornblum and Marilyn Kupetz of the TESOL Central Office for their patience and professionalism; Ellen Garshick for her insightful editorial assistance; and, most of all, our TESOL colleagues around the world who so graciously shared their ideas.

Introduction

There are many English language teachers who feel uncomfortable about presenting "the arts" in the classroom. Although Noam Chomsky resists giving advice to language teachers, he has said on various occasions that we should surround learners with the best examples of language available. For many of us, "the best" includes literature. Such an approach works very well for most teachers. By integrating the arts, specifically literature, into our teaching, we give our students excellent opportunities to express themselves in the target culture. Herbert Marcuse, the philosopher, says, "Art cannot change the world, but it can contribute to changing the consciousness and drives of the men and women who could change the world" (in Kushner, 1994). It is time to treat our students as the kind of people who can change the world.

There is an old adage that studying literature is good for one's general personal development, that it makes one a well-rounded person. There is no doubt that the study of literature encourages imagination and creativity. Many people agree that the ability to be imaginative is more important than the ability to memorize formulae. In fact, studying literature is just as important for engineers and physicists as it is for artists.

Most teachers agree that authentic language such as literature is a welcome addition to the classroom. Unfortunately many examples of English literature are simply too difficult for intermediate and low intermediate students, so publishers have simplified literary works to make them accessible to this type of student. A number of teachers are not happy with this simplification; they feel it often distorts and even destroys the original beauty of the work. As it happens, most of the lessons in this book refer to unsimplified literary texts.

Contributors to this volume have come up with original and exciting ways to incorporate literature into the language classroom. The ideas represented in the contributions range from lessons for young children to ideas for lessons for students in graduate school. The authors of these lessons range from students in graduate school to leaders in the field with well-known names. Geographically, the range is enormous. There are contributions from teachers all over the world.

We have divided the book into four chapters: Prose, Poetry, Drama, and A Mixed Bag. Teachers can find ideas that refer to literature published all over the world and from the past and the present. The selections in A Mixed Bag incorporate prose, poetry, drama, or all three. Each selection is marked as to whether it is suitable for beginners to advanced learners. Contributors also suggest whether the ideas are appropriate for children, adolescents, or adults.

All the lessons in this book will challenge the intellects of our students and help them practice the English that they already know. By using literature, we can teach the language and at the same time, we can teach them many other things about the world. Let's introduce our students to the best that English can offer them—literature.

References and Further Reading

Carter, R., & Long, M. L. (1991). *Teaching literature.* London: Longman.

Collie, J., & Slater, S. (1987). *Literature in the language classroom.* Cambridge: Cambridge University Press.

Duff, A., & Maley, A. (1990). *Literature.* Oxford: Oxford University Press.

Greenwood, J. (1988). *Class readers.* Oxford: Oxford University Press.

Hill, J. (1986). *Using literature in language teaching.* London: Macmillan.

Kushner, T. (1994). *Angels in America* (Program Notes). Performance in Johannesburg, South Africa.

Lazar, G. (1993). *Literature and language teaching.* Cambridge: Cambridge University Press.

Smith, S. (1984). *The theater arts and the teaching of languages.* New York: Addison-Wesley.

Wessels, C. (1987). *Drama.* Oxford: Oxford University Press.

Users' Guide to Activities

Part I: Prose
Bennett, J. L.: The Plot Thickens 4
Buell, M. Z.: Everyone Has a Different Story:
   A Reading and Performance Project. 6
Butler, L.: A Cooperative Learning Approach to Novels 9
Chang, J. H.: Story Rewriting. 15
Díaz Maggioli, G. H.: The Story Game 17
Díaz Maggioli, G. H.: All the World's a Stage 19
Díaz Maggioli, G. H.: Never-Ending Stories 21
Díaz Maggioli, G. H.: Wooden Characters 23
Gajdusek, L., Balason, D., Murphy, J.: Getting Psyched to
   Read Novels 25
Hess, N.: Talk Back to the Movies 30
Hetherton, G.: *Animal Farm* Revisited 35
Hetherton, G.: Video View: Give and Take 37
Lazar, G.: Who's Telling the Story?. 38
Malkina, N.: Fun With Storytelling 41
Sarmecanic, L.: Making Meaning Through a Dialectical Journal. 43
Schulte, C. G.: Just Picture It 46
Sharkey, J.: Who Did What When? 48
Tandlichová, E.: Finding a Description in a Short Story 51
Vandrick, S.: Quote/Unquote 55
Whiteson, V.: Multicultural Ideas 58
Winer, L.: All-Purpose Dialogue Journal Preview Questions 60

Part II: Poetry
Butler, L.: Using Borrowed Lines. 66
George, D.: Poem Charades. 68
Hetherton, G.: Poetic Slips 69

Hetherton, G.: The Numbers Game: 5-7-5 71
Humphries, R.: Rhyme Time 73
Lie, A.: Act It Out 75
Meloni, C., Matthews, C.: The Music of Poetry:
    Poe's "Annabel Lee" 76
Schulte, C. G.: What Is a Poem (Not)? 80
Schulte, C. G: Note to a Plum Thief 82
Solé, D.: Poetry for Pronunciation, Pronunciation for Poetry 84

Part III : Drama

Anderson, M.: Acting Is Becoming 90
Baker, M., Isbell, K.: The Lover, the Boss, and the Mother 92
Baker, M.: The Meeting 94
Barfield, A.: Creative Acts: A Workshop Approach 96
Beniston, F.: *West Side Story:* A Lesson 100
Butler, L.: Characters Come to Life 104
Couch, P. : Interaction With Literature Via
    Student-Produced Videos 106
Gardner, D., Miller, L.: Words in Action. 109
Hetherton, G.: Silent Scene 110
Levikoff, R. E.: Playing With Narratives 112
Mansour, W.: Append a Scene 114
Mansour, W.: Playwrite and Learn English 116
Miller, L.: Acting It Out 117
Murphy, J. : Teaching Pronunciation Dramatically. 119
Root, C., Dumicich, J.: Reader's Theater: A Primer on
    Pronunciation 123
Sharkey, J.: Lennie, What Were You Going to Do With
    All Those Rabbits? 125
Whiteson, V.: Writing a Scene From a Play 127

Part IV: A Mixed Bag

Abdel Khalek, N. A.: Young Playwrights 131
Butler, L.: Jumpstart Discussion With Think/Pair/Share 133
Davis, L.: When a Pig Builds a Bungalow: Working With Titles 135

Hess, N.: Put a Ring Around the Thing 138
Hess, N.: Walk For a Good Talk 141
Hetherton, G.: Choral Chant 144
Schulte, C. G.: Words They Can Keep 146
Schulte, C. G.: Connections 149
Wilcoxon, H.: Thinking Through Metaphors 152

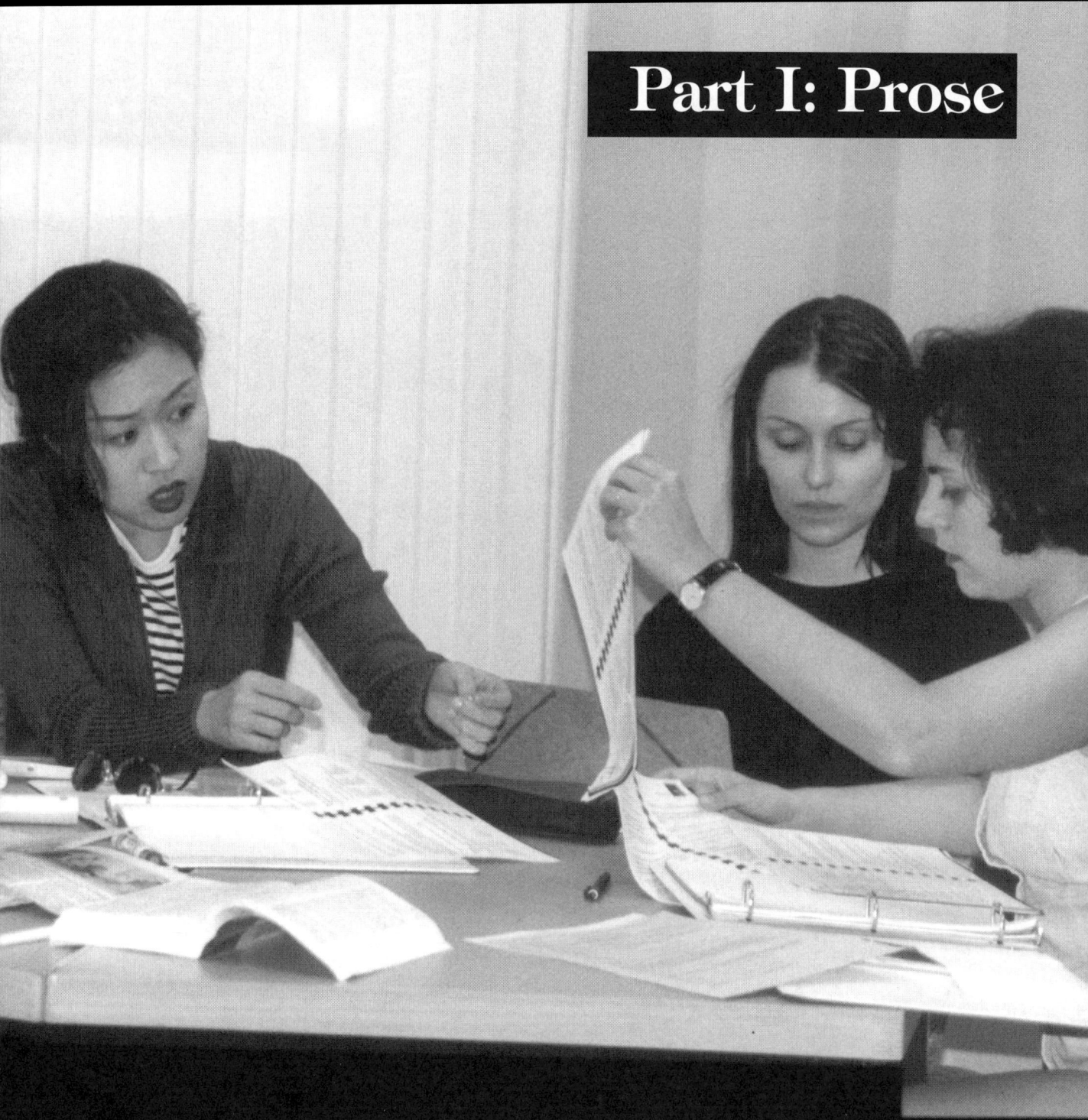
Part I: Prose

Left to right: Jee Hae Kwon, Crystel Kohler, and Soraia Martins at Eurocentres, Alexandria, Virginia USA.

Introduction

The most important consideration when choosing prose to study in the TESOL classroom is that both the teacher and the class enjoy the selection. Does the selection have to be great literature? Certainly not. It is, however, important to pick material that will ultimately produce good conversation and writing. Choose readings that are a little too difficult for your class rather than too easy. Be especially careful not to insult their intelligence with childish books and stories. Most experienced teachers start out gradually: short stories; then extracts from novels; finally a novel. Look for a novel with short chapters, uncomplicated language, and universal themes. I have had great success with Alice Walker's *The Color Purple*, for example.

Part I of this volume contains a wealth of ideas for using prose with just about any class.

The Plot Thickens

Levels
Intermediate +

Aims
Understand literary concepts through student-generated stories

Class Time
Variable

Resources
Roberts and Jacobs (1987)

This activity engages students in the active exploration of the idea of plot (which includes actions and their causation) and may be expanded to include other elements of literary analysis, especially characters and setting.

Procedure

1. Divide the class into small groups of three to four students.
2. Introduce E. M. Forster's illustration of plot: "The king died, and then the queen died" (Roberts & Jacobs, 1987, p. 88).
3. After pointing out the significance of adding "of grief" to the second clause in the example above ("The king died, and then the queen died of grief."), write the words *the king died* on one side of the chalkboard and *the queen died* on the other half of the chalkboard.
4. Ask students to consider for a moment how the king and queen died.
5. Call on individual students to describe the cause of only one death.
6. Record students' responses on the board, as students continue to brainstorm possible causes.
7. Thicken the plot as you go along, asking detailed questions or adding whatever comments are necessary to stimulate students' creative juices.
8. Ask students to discuss and develop the plots further in small-group discussions.
9. As homework, assign students to create their own short story about the king and queen and be prepared to tell it to their group in the next class. At that time, have each group select one person to tell one version of the story to the class.

Caveats and Options

1. Ask students to write their stories and have small groups analyze them in class.
2. Select a story that students have already read, and ask them to discuss its plot in small groups and report their conclusions to the class.
3. Students' associations with the words *king* and *queen* may vary with their cultural backgrounds. Asking students to examine this issue may lead to a greater appreciation of literature in general and of the way culture can influence the creative process.

References and Further Reading

Roberts, E. V., & Jacobs, H. E. (1987). *Literature: An introduction to reading and writing*. Englewood Cliffs, NJ: Prentice Hall.

Contributor

Janet L. Bennett is an Instructor at Kansai Gaidai in Osaka, Japan. She has also taught ESOL in Germany, China, Taiwan, and the United States.

Everyone Has a Different Story: A Reading and Performance Project

Levels
Intermediate +; young adult or university students

Aims
Read and present material to the class

Class Time
5–6 hours

Preparation Time
Variable

Resources
Several short stories a little below or just at the students' comprehension level, preferably related to a common theme (see References and Further Reading)
Video camera

In this project, groups read stories that other groups do not read. Each student reads a story independently, and students who have read the same story decide how to turn the story into either a play or a puppet show for the class. By acting out the scenes, learners develop a deeper understanding of the characters, issues, and themes and experiment with ways of expressing complex ideas.

Procedure

1. Select three or four stories that are related to a common theme. Topics that have come up in class discussion work well. Look for stories that have several characters so that everyone in a group has a speaking role.
2. Divide the students into groups of seven or eight, or let them create their own groups. Assign one of the stories to each group.
3. Tell the students to individually read and summarize their stories, making notes on the plot, characters, setting, and theme. This can be done as homework.
4. Have the students share their summaries and their impressions with group members who have read the same story. Then ask the groups to decide what will be important to present and what can be cut. Advise the groups as needed.
5. Let the groups decide whether they will produce a play or a puppet show and have them distribute roles as they see fit. Offer suggestions on how to expand or modify small roles, divide narration, or introduce the story so that all group members have a speaking role.

Encourage equal contribution to all aspects of the performance by requiring that performances include
- an introduction of characters and setting, along with an explanation of any new and important vocabulary
- the story itself, told in an interesting and clear way
- questions for the audience to discuss, including questions about both the story itself and the theme

6. Set aside all or part of several classes for students to modify scripts, gather props and materials, and rehearse. Meet with each group during these sessions to check understanding of the stories, answer questions about procedures, and coach actors on their deliveries. (As rehearsal sessions progress, groups will probably become more independent, allowing you to work on specific problems as they come up.) Encourage groups to rehearse outside of class as well.
7. Schedule student performances. Have a student operate the video camera so that you can join the audience to watch the performances.
8. Use the videotapes to evaluate student work on the project. Have students give feedback on the project. (See the Appendix.)
9. If students want to watch their videotapes, arrange for them to do so in an informal setting.

Caveats and Options

1. This project works best if the students know each other well and have already given presentations in class.
2. If there are not enough students for the roles, have some students play more than one role. If there are too many students, some groups may opt to have one role played by more than one student. This will have to be made clear to the audience.
3. There may be enough characters for the students, but the female-to-male ratio may cause a problem. In some cases, characters can change gender without affecting the story. If this is not possible, have women play men or men play women, but again, make sure the audience knows who is who. Some students may want to play the opposite sex for comic effect.
4. Question-and-answer sessions may be a little awkward. Be prepared to step in to help with discussion or explanations. Encourage discussion on the theme once all the performances are complete.

References and Further Reading

Mansfield, K. (1993). The doll's house. In C. G. Thornley (Ed.), *Outstanding short stories* (Simplified ed.) (pp. 38-45). Essex, England: Longman.

Mundahl, J. (1993). The poor woman's gift. In J. Mundahl (Ed.), *Tales of courage, tales of dreams* (pp. 52-56). New York: Addison-Wesley.

Sieruta, P. (1995). Being alive. In R. Cormier (Ed.), *Crossroads: Classic themes in young adult literature* (pp. 106-123). Glenview, IL: Scott Foresman.

Appendix: Story Presentation Survey

In December, you prepared performances based on different stories. This involved reading a story; discussing the plot, theme, setting, and characters; and using this information to make a play or puppet show. Please share your thoughts and opinions on this project.

1. In your opinion, what was the purpose of this project?
2. How did you feel about the reading section of this project? What did you do to understand the story well? What, if any, reading skills were improved by working on this project? Also note how you felt about reading something that not all your classmates read.
3. How do you feel about your speaking part in this presentation? Comment on working with a group and your own participation. What, if any, speaking skills were improved by working on this project?
4. How do you feel about your classmates' performances? Could you understand most of the stories you watched? Would you be interested in reading the stories they presented?
5. Circle the words that you agree with:
    I think we spent too much/enough/too little time on this project.
    I think the project was/was not a valuable use of class time.
    I would like/would not like to do this sort of project again.
6. How can the project be improved?

Please feel free to add any additional comments.

Contributor

Marcia Z. Buell teaches ESL at Kansai Foreign Language University in Japan. She has also taught ESL in China, Hungary, and the United States.

A Cooperative Learning Approach to Novels

Levels
Intermediate +;
secondary +

Aims
Read novels in English
Enhance comprehension and enjoyment of reading
Think critically and take responsibility for learning

Class Time
Variable

Preparation Time
Variable

Resources
Novel appropriate to the level and age of the class

Ongoing cooperative learning (CL) groups to discuss a novel will increase student involvement in the reading and interaction in class. Students find they cannot read in a perfunctory way in the expectation that you will explain the novel to them. Instead they face each other, help each other, and learn from having to articulate their own ideas. You can step into a coaching role while students work to gain understanding of the text.

Procedure

1. Create heterogeneous groups of three to five students. Try to balance them in terms of academic proficiency, English skills, age, gender, and language and cultural background. These groups will work together for the duration of the novel.
2. Plan for evaluation and reward to promote both group interdependence and individual accountability. Possibilities include
   - requiring portfolios based on the novel that include student writing (e.g., essays and journal entries) plus work done by the group and the student's reflections on the CL approach
   - basing grades on both a group presentation and individual achievement (e.g., homework completion, journals, essays)
   - having students assess their own and each other's contributions to their group
   - giving students bonus points when all members of their team achieve a certain score on a test on the novel
3. Talk with the class about the reasons for reading novels and for reading as a class the one you are assigning. (See References and Further Reading for suggestions.) Outline the plan for reading the novel—the homework assignments, the nature of the work in class, and the means of assessment. Provide handouts describing the roles

the students will take in their groups and a (tentative) schedule for completing the novel.
4. Go over expressions useful in asking for clarification, politely disagreeing, checking for comprehension, providing encouragement, and so on to highlight the language and behaviors needed for group success.
5. Look at the novel with the class. Examine and discuss the front and back covers and any introductory information given about the author. Use open-ended questions, true/false statements, free writing, and so on to elicit what students know and believe about the time and place that will be the setting for the novel.
6. Assign the portion of the novel to be read for the next class. Hand out the preliminary questions to be answered about this reading. Basic comprehension questions help students judge whether they have understood the main points about the setting, characters, and plot; writing their answers helps them consolidate their knowledge of the story and sort out their thoughts about it. Include questions that ask about personal opinions and relevant experiences. Encourage students to write down any questions they want to ask you. (See the Appendix for examples.)
7. At the next class,
   - go over some or all of the homework questions to lay a foundation for CL group discussions, collecting the papers later, or
   - collect the homework papers and scan them (while students begin work in their groups) for any major misconceptions that you want to address immediately.
8. Have students gather in their groups and choose roles for that day's discussion. (Provide each group with a folder in which to keep group papers and record their roles.) There will need to be a *facilitator,* someone who will stimulate discussion, keep the group focused, and encourage participation by all group members.

   Choose three or four other roles for students to take on in their groups. Possible roles include
   - *timekeeper,* who makes sure the group progresses toward completion of their task within the time you have allowed

- *summarizer*, who sums up group answers to each question
- *checker*, who makes sure that all group members understand and, if consensus is required, are in agreement
- *recorder*, who writes down the group's response(s) to each question
- *observer*, who keeps track of how the group is functioning
- *spokesperson*, who reports to the full class on the group's discussion.

9. Give each group one copy of the discussion questions for the day. These questions should require students to analyze what they have read, to find support in the text for the opinions they give, and to use the text as a springboard for debating issues of interest to them. Let students know that some questions have one good answer they must discover and agree on; others may have more than one good answer. (See the Appendix for suggestions and examples of discussion questions.) Have the students complete their work together by considering how they have functioned as a group.
10. While students are at work in their groups, circulate among them to monitor group functioning and serve as a resource: clarifying questions, reading aloud key passages, providing encouragement, and so on.
11. Have the full class reassemble. For each discussion question, ask one spokesperson to report on the discussion in the group; then ask the other spokespersons how their groups' responses to that question were similar or different. (Begin with a different spokesperson on each question.) Open the floor to comments and questions about the novel from all students. Collect the papers from each group.
12. Give the reading assignment and homework questions for the following class.
13. At the following class, allow time for the groups to read and discuss any comments you have written on their papers before going on with their next discussion.
14. Elicit feedback from students on a regular basis (both in conversation and in writing) on their experiences with this approach to reading the novel.

Caveats and Options

1. If students do not know each other well, promote team building before beginning work on the novel by setting up an enjoyable activity for students to do in their groups.
2. Ask students to keep reading journals in which they record aspects of the novel that strike them and their reactions to those aspects. In their groups, have them share what they have written.
3. Some students will read ahead in the novel. Encourage them in this, but tell them that in their groups they must focus on the current task and not reveal to others what lies ahead in the story.
4. Don't let the groups get bogged down in composing their answers to the discussion questions. Urge them to write brief answers; the spokesperson can go into greater detail.
5. Make clear to the students that when they are absent, they must consult their teammates to find out what they missed.
6. Maintain a careful balance between individual and team rewards. There needs to be an incentive for stronger students to invest in the learning of weaker students, but one student's poor performance cannot penalize the rest of the team.
7. Vary CL group discussion with activities such as role plays and reader's theater. (See related activities in Part III: Drama.)

References and Further Reading

Steinbeck, J. (1937). *Of mice and men*. New York: Viking.

For information on cooperative learning:

Cooperative Learning and College Teaching Newsletter. Available from New Forums Press, Inc., 1722 Cimarron Plaza, Stillwater, OK 74075.

Johnson, D. W., & Johnson, R. T. (1991). *Learning together and alone: Cooperative, competitive, and individualistic learning* (3rd ed.). Boston: Allyn & Bacon.

Johnson, D. W., Johnson, R. T., & Smith, K. A. (1991). *Cooperative learning: Increasing college faculty instructional productivity*. (ASHE-ERIC Higher Education Report No. 4). Washington, DC: The George Washington University.

For lists of novels recommended for ESOL students:

Brown, D. (1988). *A world of books: An annotated reading list for ESL/EFL students* (2nd ed.). Washington, DC: TESOL.

Appendix: Sample Questions and Activities

Brown, D. (1994). *Books for a small planet: A multicultural-intercultural bibliography for young English language learners*. Alexandria, VA: TESOL.

MacGowan-Gilhooly, A. (1993). *Achieving fluency in English: A whole-language book* (2nd ed.). Dubuque, IA: Kendall/Hunt.

In homework questions, focus on the basics: Who? What? Where? Avoid yes/no questions unless students are asked to explain their answers. Ask students to react to and make predictions about the story. Where appropriate, ask about students' own experiences that relate to incidents and ideas in the story.

In their groups, students can handle more challenging questions, such as ones that ask *Why? How are ___ and ___ similar/different? What would happen if? What does ___ mean when he/she says ___? How does ___ affect ___? Do you agree with the following statement: ___? Why or why not?* Students can also compare any predictions and reactions they wrote for homework.

The following are examples of questions about the novel *Of Mice and Men* (Steinbeck, 1937).

Homework Questions for Chapter 5:
1. What has happened to Lennie's puppy?
2. What does Curley's wife talk to Lennie about?
3. What happens to her?
4. Where is Lennie going?
5. What are the men planning to do?
6. Carlson claims Lennie has stolen his gun. Do you believe him? Why or why not?
7. Write any questions you have about this chapter.

CL Group Discussion Questions for Chapter 5
1. Do you agree with the following statement?
    Curley's wife is trying to seduce Lennie; she wants him to make love to her.
   Explain your answers.

2. a. List three different things that might happen to Lennie that are discussed by the men.
   b. Considering these possibilities, what should George do?
3. Whose fault is the killing? Decide how much responsibility each person has for what happened: Lennie, Curley's wife, Curley, George. Rank them from most to least responsible, and prepare to explain your reasoning to the rest of the class.

Group Processing
1. What was something each group member did today that was helpful?
2. What is something each group member can do to make the group better next time?

Contributor

Linda Butler teaches ESL, writes, and consults in Massachusetts, in the United States. She is the creator of The ESOL Reader's Companion *series (McGraw-Hill).*

Story Rewriting

Levels
Any

Aims
Increase reading, writing, and speaking abilities

Class Time
Variable

Preparation Time
10 minutes

Resources
Tales, fables, short stories

This activity offers a creative way of understanding the process of writing. It may raise students' awareness of some important elements involved in writing.

Procedure

1. Distribute a one- to two-page story.
2. Read and discuss the story with the whole class.
3. Ask the students to form several groups. Each group should decide its audience (e.g., adults, teenagers, or small children); purpose (e.g., to inform, entertain, or persuade); and tone (e.g., serious, ironic, or humorous).
4. Have each group work as a team to rewrite the story. Every student can and should contribute ideas during the writing process, but each student should be assigned a duty—to check spelling, grammar, punctuation, usage, line of development, for example.
5. Make corrections and suggestions on the new versions of the story.
6. Have students act out the story.

Caveats and Options

1. Encourage imagination while you emphasize the logical development.
2. Point out the merits of the rewritten stories before you comment on the parts that need to be improved.
3. The story "Little Red Riding Hood" works well.

References and Further Reading

Gillespie, S., Singleton, R., & Becker, R. (1989). *The writer's craft* (2nd ed.). London: Scott Foresman.

Contributor

Jane H. Chang is Associate Professor of EFL in the Department of Foreign Languages and Literature, National Chung Cheng University in Taiwan, Republic of China.

The Story Game

Levels
Beginning +

Aims
Voice opinions about a literary piece

Class Time
45 minutes

Preparation Time
15 minutes

Resources
Storyboard
Dice
Question cards

This activity allows all learners in a class to voice their opinions about a story, review the facts, and pose questions about obscure points in it. It is geared mainly toward tactile/kinesthetic students and is valuable in helping visual learners speak. It frees the teacher and allows cooperative group work, emphasizing such strategies as questioning for clarification, cooperating, reviewing, and inferencing.

Procedure

1. Before class, review the last story or literary piece you worked with and prepare 10 cards, each containing a question that requires students to give factual information about the literary piece (Fact questions, showing a magnifying glass), their opinion about it (Opinion questions, showing either a microphone or a loudspeaker) and blank cards depicting a question mark.
2. After the students have read the piece of literature, ask them to form groups and distribute the storyboards and the sets of cards (see Appendix). Appoint a secretary in each group.
3. Instruct students to roll the dice and start moving along the board. Whenever they land on a square with a picture, have them pick up a card and either answer the factual or opinion question or ask the rest of the group a question. If the question cannot be answered by any group member, have the secretary record it for a later stage.
4. Allow all students to complete a circle around the board. After they have all finished, ask learners to write their unanswered questions on the board while you leave the room for 5 minutes.
5. When you return, ask each student to take three pieces of paper and try to answer the questions. Read these answers out loud to the rest of the group.

6. If any of the questions has not been answered, guide students toward discovering the answer or making a conclusion.

Appendix: Storyboard and Sample Cards

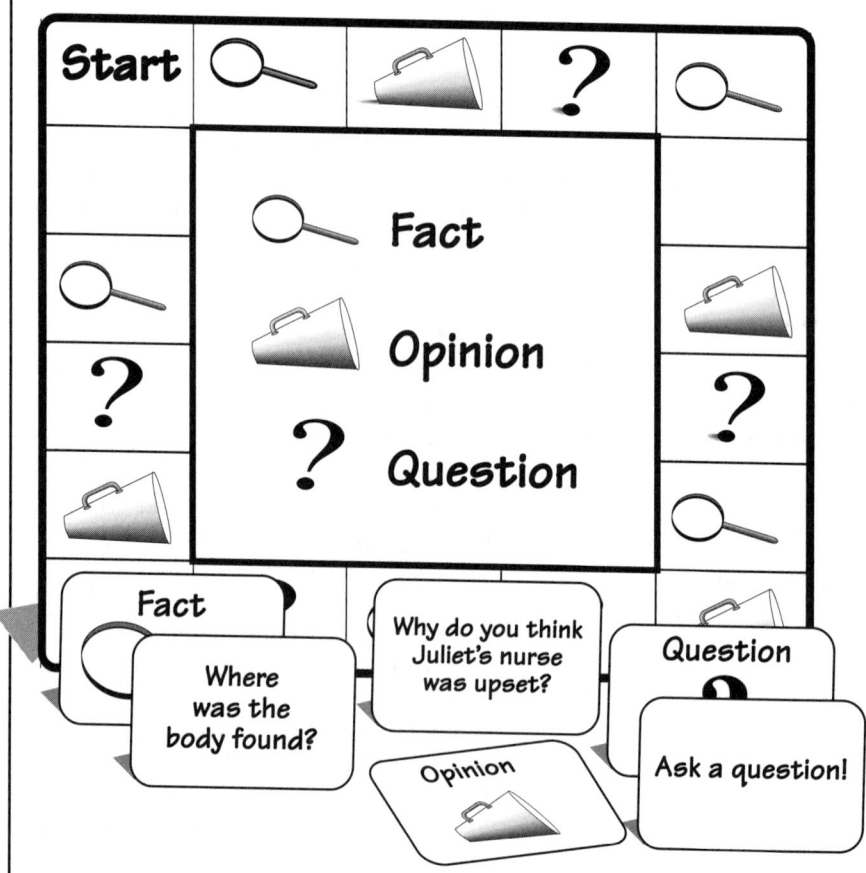

Contributor

Gabriel H. Díaz Maggioli is a life-long learner from his own learners as well as a teacher, teacher educator, and materials writer in Montevideo, Uruguay.

All the World's a Stage . . .

Levels
Intermediate +

Aims
Perceive the multitude of meanings in a literary piece

Class Time
About 50 minutes

Preparation Time
None

Resources
Copies of a game board
Dice
Copies of a literary work

Any piece of literature is a kaleidoscope that depicts all human traits in one way or another. This activity helps learners reflect on the hidden meanings and symbols of a story, play, or novel while voicing their opinions. Because of its design, it helps all kinds of learners and fosters cooperation in the class. It also takes the burden off the analysis of literary pieces and allows students to apply strategies such as imagery and inferencing naturally.

Procedure

1. As you finish reading a work of literature, instruct students to sit in groups of four to six and bring their copy of the work with them.
2. Appoint functionaries within each group: a timekeeper, an artist (who records important information), an encourager (also known as cheerleader), and a reporter (who will later speak to the rest of the class).
3. Give each group a literary board (see the Appendix) and a die and tell them to roll the die and advance around the board by elaborating on the element in each square on which they land with reference to the work of literature. Set a time limit of 2 minutes per turn. Have students who fail to respond to one of the cues on the board miss a turn. The aim of the game is to reach the FINISH square.
4. Bring the class together. Have the reporters from the different groups give their group's conclusions and remarks.

Caveats and Options

Have learners do this activity as an end-of-term assignment to spot similar themes in the different pieces of literature read in the course.

Appendix: Literary Board

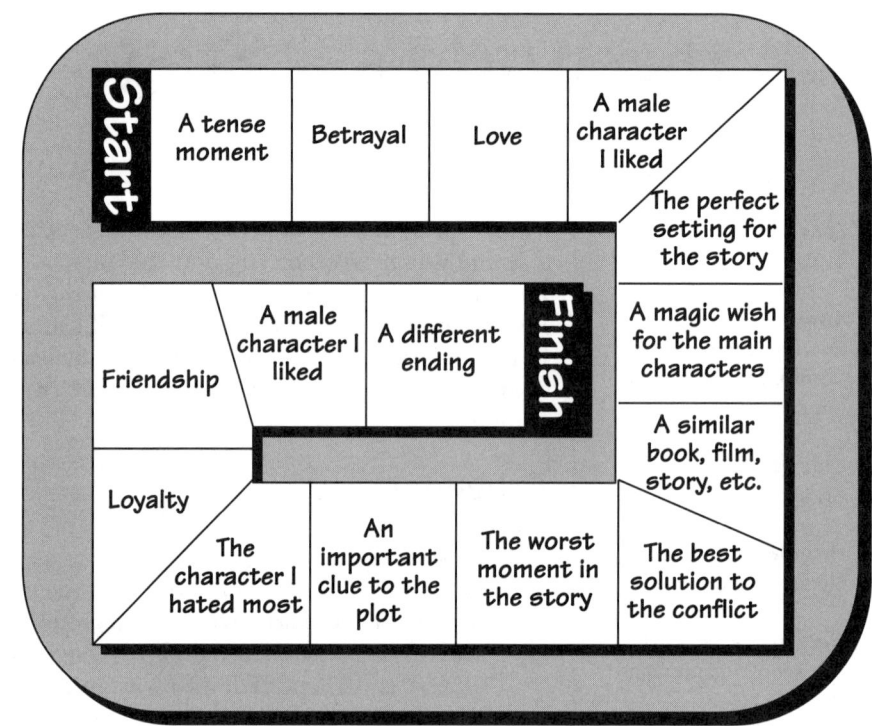

Contributor

Gabriel H. Díaz Maggioli is a life-long learner from his own learners as well as a teacher, teacher educator, and materials writer in Montevideo, Uruguay.

Never-Ending Stories

Levels
High beginning +

Aims
Understand text by relating literature to the here and now

Class Time
About 20 minutes

Preparation Time
None

Resources
None

Handling a literary classic in class can be discouraging for students who fail to relate the masterpiece to the reality around them. In making the story current by means of different props and by interacting with their peers, the institution, and the outside world, the students can make the characters, setting, and story their own and start enjoying and understanding it. In Freire's (1970) words, "Reading the world precedes reading the word" (p. 42).

Procedure

1. After having read a literary classic in class, ask the students to dissect it into component parts such as theme, main male characters, main female character, main child character, secondary characters, settings, feelings, and so on.
2. Write the list on the board. For each item ask groups of students to bring to class and display
   - a painting
   - a song
   - some graffiti
   - other material from outside the classroom

   that epitomizes each component. Alternatively, ask the students to suggest things from content areas, such as a historical character or event, an animal, a chemical element, a law of physics, or a mathematical equation. Insist that the important point is to justify their choices and not just to bring the prop. Make sure students know why they have chosen their props.

3. After students have brought all their samples and displayed them, pair the groups and hold a 5-minute argument session in which one group tries to challenge the other group about their choices, always supporting their challenges with sound reasons.
4. Ask the rest of the class to vote for the best argument and element.

References and Further Reading

Freire, P. (1970). *Pedagogía del oprimido.* Montevideo, Uruguay: Siglo XXI Editores.

Contributor

Gabriel H. Díaz Maggioli is a life-long learner from his learners as well as a teacher, teacher educator, and materials writer in Montevideo, Uruguay.

Wooden Characters

Levels
Beginning +

Aims
Make and test hypotheses about plot, characters, and theme

Class Time
15 minutes the first day
A few minutes on subsequent days

Preparation Time
None

Resources
Box of Cuisenaire rods
Table

Literature appears most of the time as an abstract phenomenon in the students' minds. Finding ways of making a story concrete helps improve comprehension. This activity focuses on ways to reinforce the different learning modalities and allows all kinds of learners to participate. It is also useful in exercising strategies such as deducing, inferencing, predicting, and using background knowledge together with employing action and imagery.

Procedure

1. Before starting the reading of a literary selection, briefly inform the class of the general theme and plot of the story. Also mention the number of characters, dividing them into main/secondary and protagonist/antagonist. Write these items on the chalkboard and ask students to suggest adjectives to describe the characters, settings, plot, theme, and other elements.
2. Present the box of Cuisenaire rods and invite the students to "map" their predictions about the story on the table. Have each student contribute an element. Always ask for a reason when students choose a rod. For example, in dealing with *Macbeth*, tell them it is a tragedy involving two kings. A student may choose two orange rods (the longest ones in the set) to represent them because they are important.
3. Allow students to create settings and build structures using the rods.
4. As the reading of the story progresses, devote 5 or 10 minutes to having students add suggestions to change the initial story rod map by adding, substituting, or deleting elements.
5. Have one or two students in the class keep track of the different maps so they can compare the predictions and expand on them.

6. After the reading is complete, have students copy and label the story rod map, which will serve as a quick reference. Have them include character, story, and setting traits and characteristics alongside their names.

Contributor

Gabriel H. Díaz Maggioli is a life-long learner from his own learners as well as a teacher, teacher educator, and materials writer in Montevideo, Uruguay.

Getting Psyched to Read Novels

Levels
College bound and college enrolled

Aims
Explore and apply abstract concepts from a content course

Class Time
1 hour of class, four times per term

Preparation Time
Less than 1 hour

Resources
Copies of a novel

In this activity, structured study questions guide students to read and become involved with the characters and conflicts of a novel. The teacher exploits this involvement to explore and apply to the novel the abstract and often difficult concepts of more traditional reading content, such as psychology. As they strive to apply the academic concepts appropriately, the students gain an understanding of these concepts and insight into the world of the novel. As they answer the study questions at home, the students begin their personal interaction with the novel. This prepares them for animated and focused small-group discussion during the class.

Procedure

1. Assign the chosen novel to each student at the beginning of the term.
2. At least a week before each planned small-group discussion, assign the study questions (see the Appendix).
3. Have students meet in small groups to discuss the novel in terms of their responses to the study questions. During this time, visit the groups and monitor their progress, verify comprehension, and make comments and suggestions.
4. Within these small groups, on worksheets, or both, have students choose academic concepts from material recently covered in the content course (psychology, in this case) and find examples in their novels.
5. As culminating activities
   - Have students give panel presentations during which each group presents academic concepts (e.g., for psychology, defense mecha-

nisms, stages of moral reasoning, locus of control) as they play out in the novel.
- Have students write reports that present the novel in terms of the concepts being explored.

Caveats and Options

1. Assign different novels to different students to stimulate more challenging and communicative interaction. Instead of focusing on a single novel during small-group discussion, assign one reader of each novel to each group. Have each group member fill the information gap for the rest of the group, using the study questions as a springboard for discussion. Suggestions for psychology content courses include *Walking Across Egypt* (Edgerton, 1993), *Flowers for Algernon* (Keyes, 1975), *A Separate Peace* (Knowles, 1975), and *Of Mice and Men* (Steinbeck, 1937/1992).
2. The handouts in the Appendix, which are specific to psychology content courses, can be adapted for any academic discipline or novel.

References and Further Reading

Edgerton, C. (1993). *Walking across Egypt.* New York: Ballantine Books.
Keyes, D. (1975). *Flowers for Algernon.* New York: Bantam Books.
Knowles, J. (1975). *A separate peace.* New York: Bantam Books.
Steinbeck, J. (1992). *Of mice and men.* New York: Penguin Books. (Original work published 1937)

Appendix

Worksheets for *A Separate Peace* (Knowles, 1975)

Section 1

1. Who is the author? When was the novel first published?
2. Read the first page. Who or what is this page about? Do you think the book will be mainly about this person or thing? Why or why not? Where does the action of the first page take place?

Now read the first section of your book (pp. 1–52).

3. Who is the narrator, or what is the point of view? Write a sentence that gives evidence about who the narrator is. If the narrator is a character in the story, describe him/her: age? gender? profession? physical appearance? personality? etc.
4. List the other main characters and their relationships to the main character.
5. Summarize what happens in the first section of the story.
6. What questions do you have about the book so far? For example, was there a part where you did not understand what was happening? Was there a concept or idea that you'd like to know more about? Write any words that you did not know—choose words that seem important for understanding the situation. Write the word and then write what you think the word means or what kind of thing it talks about.
7. Draw a time line to show the year of the first sentence of the book and the year of the main action of the story. Add any historical events that you know about that fit on your time line.

Section 2

Read the second section of your novel (pp. 53-94).

1. Identify each of the main characters in relation to at least one other character. What new things have you learned about these characters that you did not know about them in the first section of the novel?
2. Summarize the situation at the beginning of the second section.
3. List the main events in this section.
4. Scan to find quotes that show how much time has passed from the beginning of the book to the point where you are now and list them.
5. Think of three adjectives to describe the main character and support your choices with quotes or evidence from the novel.
6. The writer probably assumes readers are familiar with certain cultural issues. Talk to a native speaker to find out more about private school mentality and "intellectual geek" vs. "dumb jock" stereotypes. How is understanding this concept important for understanding your book?

Section 3

Read the third section of your novel (pp. 95–150).

1. Identify any new characters you met in this section of the book.
2. List the main events from this section of the book.
3. List quotes that show how much time has passed from the beginning of the book to the point where you are now.
4. A theme is a generalization about human nature or human behavior. What are some themes from your novel?
5. If you haven't already finished your novel, how do you think it is going to end? If you have already finished it, were you surprised by the ending? Explain.
6. Choose two characters and analyze their social development in terms of Erik Erikson's stages of psychosocial development. What are some positive and negative sides of their development? Give at least three quotes to support your answer.
7. Choose two of Sigmund Freud's defense mechanisms and explain how a main character in your novel is exhibiting this behavior. Provide quotes to support your answer.
8. What Myers-Briggs Type Indicator personality type do you think one of your main characters would have? Explain why.

Section 4

Finish the novel.

1. List the main events from this section of the novel.
2. List quotes that show how much time has passed from the beginning of the book to the point where you are now.
3. What is the significance of the title of your novel? In other words, why do you think the novel is called *A Separate Peace*?
4. The climax of a story usually occurs close to the end and is the most important or exciting event of the story. Action in the story builds toward this turning point, and once it occurs, you can usually predict how the story will end. What was the climax of your novel? Explain why you think this was the climax.

Choose two of the following characters (Gene, Finny, Leper) to analyze in Questions 5–7.

5. Review Abraham Maslow's hierarchy of needs. Indicate the position of two characters in his hierarchy. How have they met their needs at previous levels? How are they trying to meet their needs at their current level? Explain, giving details from your novel.
6. Do the two characters have a positive or negative self-concept? High or low self-esteem? An internal or external locus of control? Explain the choices you made.

Contributors

Linda Gajdusek, Denise Balason, and Jennifer Murphy are ESL Instructors at Georgia State University, in the United States.

Talk Back to the Movies

Levels
Intermediate +

Aims
Speak, read, expand vocabulary

Class Time
45-90 minutes per session

Preparation Time
5-10 minutes before each session
2 hours for the unit

Resources
Videotape player
Videotaped/film version of a novel
Copies of the novel

This series of activities integrates text with video or film to bolster extensive reading. If used appropriately, the video helps to maintain momentum during the extensive reading of a novel.

Procedure

Before class

1. Choose an appropriate novel for your class. (See Caveats and Options for suggestions.) The novel should
   - have a clear and interesting plot line
   - possess literary value
   - have themes with universal appeal
   - have a vocabulary level that is challenging but not impossibly demanding
   - have a good video version that is fairly compatible with the text
2. Divide the novel into sections appropriate for weekly readings in your class. Three or four chapters each week is about right.
3. Write out questions that will serve as a reading guide for each unit.
4. Write summaries for the first three units.
5. Find a central theme in each reading unit. Choose one scene in the reading that clearly demonstrates the theme. Then locate the corresponding scene in the video. Or first choose an absorbing scene in the video and then look for its complementary book scene.

    For example, in Tyler's (1986) *The Accidental Tourist,* the theme of the first unit is travel. The scene chosen is an opening scene in the movie, but it does not appear until chapter 15 in the book. In this scene Macon, on his travels, meets a fat man who is his admirer.

In Class

1. Introduce the novel by telling the class a few interesting aspects of the writer's life and reasons for the great popularity of the book. If the book has an intriguing cover or jacket design, talk about it and ask students to guess what the book might be about. For example, in *The Accidental Tourist*, there is a picture of a flying armchair on the cover. Discussion might center on the usual function of an armchair and about the meaning of armchair travel.
2. Briefly describe four interesting characters from the book and write these descriptions on the board. For example, for Tyler, write (a) a man who writes travel books, (b) two women who love the same man, (c) a dog that bites, and (d) a dog trainer.
3. In small groups, have students write a story projection on what the book could possibly be about.
4. Have each group ask a spokesperson to read its plot projection out loud to the class. These are usually interesting and often amusing.
5. Present a communicative activity that touches on the personal lives of students as well as on the central theme of your first reading unit. For example, for the theme of travel in Tyler, give students thought-provoking statements relating to travel. As you read them, have students mark them with *agree, disagree*, or *not sure*. Later have students mingle cocktail party style, explaining their opinions to each other.

    Sample statements are:
    - I always put too much in my suitcase.
    - I always forget an important item.
    - When I travel I miss foods from home.
    - I get nervous when I travel.
    - I love to travel.
    - I miss my family when I travel.
    - I relax when I travel.
    - I can't sleep in strange beds.
    - I miss the smells from home.

6. As students follow in their text, read the pivotal scene from the book. Make sure that students understand who the main characters

of the scene are and how they are related to each other. Write important names on the board.
7. If there is dialogue in the scene, ask students to pair up and read the dialogue to each other.
8. Have students switch partners and read the part of dialogue that they haven't yet read. (If there is no dialogue, have students choose significant aspects of the text to read out loud.)
9. Show the scene on the video.
10. In small groups, have students talk about the difference between the text and film. Ask why the filmmaker might have chosen to leave out certain aspects of the book or why other aspects might have been changed. Elicit the differences inherent in artistic media.

    Examples are that some characters have been left out because a movie producer doesn't want to pay so many actors and that some scenes may have been put in different places for reasons of visual appeal.
11. Have students view the same segment again. This time, ask them to write down as much as possible of what one character says.
12. Have students compare notes with those who were assigned the same character.
13. Have students pair up with those who have written down what another character said, and have them reconstruct the dialogue from their notes.
14. Have students reconstruct the dialogue without looking at their notes.
15. Have students check their reconstruction with the original text in the book.
16. For homework, have students read the first three or four chapters of the book.
17. Continue with once-a-week discussions of the reading bolstered by the viewing of crucial scenes.

Caveats and Options

1. The books I have found successful are Buck (1931), Dickens (1866/1963; 1849/1984), Dreiser (1925/1981), Du Maurier (1938), Lee (1960), Steinbeck (1937/1986), and Tyler (1986). Most of these also exist in abridged versions.

2. After the first three units, students are usually completely hooked on the book and no longer need summaries.
3. Once the book is read, show the entire video—perhaps at a movie party with popcorn at someone's house.
4. On a final test, ask a question that deals with a comparison between text and video.
5. Another viewing activity is the following:
   - Divide your class into two lines. Have one line sit with backs to the screen and the other line stand facing the sitters.
   - Show a scene with the sound off. Have the standing students tell the sitting ones what is happening on the screen as images flash by.
   - Have the standing and sitting students switch places. Repeat the previous step.
   - In small groups, have students summarize what they have seen.
   - Let the students view the entire scene with the sound on.
6. Have the students watch only one character throughout all the scenes viewed and write an essay on this character.
7. Show the students a speeded-up version of the scene without sound. In small groups, have them talk about what they have seen, possibly guided by teacher questions. Then show the students the scene at normal speed.

References and Further Reading

Buck, P. (1931). *The good earth*. New York: John Day.

Dickens, C. (1950). *Great expectations* (abridged and simplified by L. Doss). Hong Kong: Longman. (Original work published 1866)

Dickens, C. (1963). *Great expectations*. New York: New American Library. (Original work published 1866)

Dickens, C. (1984). *David Copperfield*. San Francisco: Mind's Eye. (Original work published 1825)

Dreiser, T. (1981). *An American tragedy*. Franklin Center, PA: Franklin Library. (Original work published 1925)

Du Maurier, D. (1938). *Rebecca*. New York: The Book League of America.

Krashen, S. (1993). *The power of reading: Insights from the research*. Englewood, CO: Libraries Unlimited.

Lazar, G. (1993). *Literature and language teaching*. Cambridge: Cambridge University Press.

Lee, H. (1960). *To kill a mockingbird*. New York: Warner Books.

Ross, N. J. (1991). Literature and film. *ELT Journal, 42*, 8.

Steinbeck, J. (1986). *Of mice and men*. New York: Viking. (Original work published 1937)

Tyler, A. (1986). *The accidental tourist*. New York: Berkeley Publishing.

Contributor

Natalie Hess is the author of textbooks for students and teachers. She has taught students and teachers in several countries.

Animal Farm Revisited

Levels
Intermediate

Aims
Explore alternative story lines using phrases from an existing story

Class Time
30 minutes

Preparation Time
30 minutes

Resources
The novel *Animal Farm* (Orwell, 1945)
Phrase cards (one per student)

In this activity, students compose a cohesive and coherent sentence containing a phrase on a card and together create a new story. They explore the alternative story lines to determine what works, which ones are possible, and which ones are satisfying.

Procedure

1. Arrange the seats in a circle.
2. Give each student a phrase card (a card containing a phrase about one of the animals in *Animal Farm*).
3. Have all the students walk around the room, perhaps while music plays. If your students are not too inhibited, get them to move around the room in a way suggested by their phrase cards.
4. Have the students freeze on command and take seats randomly.
5. Select one student to begin the story, or start it yourself and indicate who should continue. Have each student add a sentence to the story using the phrase from the card they hold.
6. While the students are relating the tale, make note of any points of interest that you will raise when all students have contributed. For example, *How plausible is . . . ? Can you say . . . in a better, more effective way?*
7. Redistribute the cards and repeat Steps 2-6 at least once, or more often if time and enthusiasm permit.

Caveats and Options

1. Most novels and short stories can be explored in this way.
2. Record the first version of the story on cassette to make study of its strong and weak points easier. Record subsequent versions and compare them.

3. Each version should show a progression and development in language use with increasingly sophisticated verbs, adjectives, and adverbs. For example, the first version may contain simple statements, whereas the second one focuses on more creative verb use, and the third, on adjectives.
4. As a follow-up activity, have the students write their favorite version of the story.
5. Divide the class in two, with one half narrating while the other half acts out the story. Heighten the dramatic effect by using puppets or masks. Students often feel liberated behind a mask or puppet so can produce more creative and interesting work.
6. In large classes, give groups of students one card. Have one member narrate while the rest of the group acts out the story, or have half of the group speak and the others perform.
7. The students may find it interesting to study the characterization of the animals in the 1985 animated version of *Animal Farm* produced by BBC Publications.

References and Further Reading

Orwell, G. (1945). *Animal farm*. London: Martin Secker & Warburg.

Contributor

Geraldine Hetherton is an EFL Lecturer at Fukui Prefectural University, Japan, and has also taught in Europe, Africa, and the Middle East.

Video View: Give and Take

Levels
Intermediate +

Aims
Compare what an author or film director presents and what the audience sees

Class Time
30 minutes

Preparation Time
10 minutes

Resources
5-minute segment of a video

Through the process of viewing, miming, and reporting on a segment of video, the students experience the personal nature of interpretation and come to realize that what is offered in a text, written or visual, may not be the same as what the reader or viewer receives.

Procedure

1. Divide the class into three groups (A, B, and C). Arrange the seating so that A can see the screen and B and C cannot.
2. Show Group A the video segment.
3. Have Group A mime what they saw on the video for Group B. Do not let Group C hear.
4. Have Group B tell Group C what Group A mimed.
5. Show all groups the video segment. Have Group C note the differences between Group B's version and the video. Have Group C mime back the differences to Groups B and A.
6. As a class, discuss the points of interest raised by the activity.

Caveats and Options

1. Screen versions of notable novels provide much suitable material for this activity.
2. This activity can offer an interesting introduction to the study of the original text.

Contributor

Geraldine Hetherton is an EFL Lecturer at Fukui Prefectural University, Japan, and has also taught in Europe, Africa, and the Middle East.

Who's Telling the Story?

Levels
High intermediate +;
adolescent and adult
learners

Aims
Draw inferences from a
range of texts

Class Time
Variable

Preparation Time
15 minutes

Resources
Opening three or four
paragraphs from at least
two novels or short
stories written in the
first person

By studying the way in which writers use language to tell a story from a particular point of view, students can improve their overall language awareness and their ability to make intelligent interpretations.

Procedure

1. Explain to students what a narrator is.
2. Have students study the opening paragraphs of two or three different novels written in the first person.
3. Help students with any problems of grammar or vocabulary.
4. Divide students into groups and ask them to complete the chart in the Appendix.
5. When students have completed the chart, discuss their answers as a class, comparing the different interpretations of the groups. Groups should be able to justify their interpretation from evidence in the text.
6. Have the class vote on which narrator the students would like to meet and why.

Caveats and Options

1. Choose texts as different as possible in terms of style, period, and identity of the narrator. A few possible texts are listed in References and Further Reading.
2. When filling in the chart, encourage students to make well-reasoned but creative inferences.

3. When discussing the texts, refer students to aspects of the style that provide clues to the identity of the narrator, such as slang, archaisms, dialect words, and formal or informal vocabulary.
4. As a creative writing exercise, ask students to fill in the questions on the chart based on a person they know or imagine. Then have them write three or four paragraphs from the point of view of that person. Tell them to think carefully about the kind of language the person is likely to use.

References and Further Reading

Bronte, C. (1981). *Jane Eyre.* New York: Bantam Books. (Original work published 1847)

Dickens, C. (1974). *Great expectations.* Harmondsworth, England: Penguin Books. (Original work published 1866)

Fitzgerald, F. S. (1983). *The great Gatsby.* Harmondsworth, England: Penguin Books. (Original work published 1922)

Salinger, J. D. (1969). *The catcher in the rye.* Harmondsworth, England: Penguin Books. (Original work published 1951)

Tan, A. (1989). *The joy luck club.* London: Minerva.

Appendix

In groups, fill in the following chart about the narrators in the texts your teacher has given you. Guess if you need to, but guess with a reason.

	TEXT 1	TEXT 2	TEXT 3
1. How old do you think the narrator is?			
2. Is the narrator male or female?			
3. What nationality is the narrator?			
4. What job/occupation does the narrator have?			
5. What is the social status of the narrator (e.g., aristocrat, middle class, working class)?			

6. Write down five or six words or phrases to describe the character or personality of the narrator.			
7. Write down three or four words or phrases to describe the emotions of the narrator.			
8. When do you think the narrator's story was written?			

Contributor

Gillian Lazar is a freelance lexicographer, teacher trainer, and the author of Literature and Language Teaching *(Cambridge University Press, 1993). She lives in London, in the United Kingdom.*

Fun With Storytelling

Levels
Beginning; children

Aims
Develop listening
comprehension skills
Learn new vocabulary
Practice *adjective +
noun* combinations in a
story context

Class Time
10 minutes

Preparation Time
About 30 minutes

Resources
Set of pictures for every
child representing
different characters of
the story

Good storytelling for early language learners is an interactive process during which both the children and the teacher-storyteller make meaning of the story. The interaction is organized in such a way that the teacher confirms the children's predictions. Children's predictions can be nonverbal for the first stage of the storytelling session; this helps them actively participate during the storytelling.

Procedure

1. Give each child a set of pictures corresponding to the characters in the story.
2. Have the children put the pictures in front of them in a row.
3. Ask the children to listen attentively and help you tell the story, showing what they think is the appropriate picture when you pause.
4. Tell the story and pause where necessary. Have the children hold up a picture during the pause. If possible, address every child, saying "right" or "wrong" to the picture. Say the word corresponding to the picture if the child holds up the right picture.
5. Have all the children put aside the right picture after each pause.
6. Continue until the children have put aside all the pictures.
7. Have the children say all the names for the pictures that they have put aside.
8. Have the children mix up their pictures and then arrange them in the order they appeared in the story.
9. Have one child name the picture while the others say "right" or "wrong."
10. Have all the children say the names for the picture again.

Caveats and Options

1. Encourage active participation.
2. Use a short and repetitive story.
3. The best type of story to use is one in which the character faces a problem and walks from one character to another trying to solve the problem, like *Who Will Be My Mother?* (Cowley, 1986).
4. Using the same plot structure, use sets of pictures to introduce new characters into the story (e.g., substitute *a cow* for *a monkey*) and practice adjective + noun combinations (e.g., substitute *a blue cow* for *a cow*).

References and Further Reading

Cowley, J. (1986). *Who will be my mother?* (programme designed by J. Melser). London: Shortland.

Contributor

Natasha Malkina, doctoral student at Hertzen Pedagogical University of Russia in St. Petersburg, Russia, is the author of many articles on teaching EFL to preschool children.

Making Meaning Through a Dialectical Journal

Levels
Intermediate +

Aims
Explore the meaning of a novel by entering into a dialogue with the text

Class Time
50 minutes

Preparation Time
30 minutes

Resources
Novel of your choice

This activity helps students become engaged in a novel by showing them a way of investigating how what they read connects with their own views and experience of life.

Procedure

1. Ask the students to come to class having read the first chapter only of the novel you have selected for study. (See References and Further Reading for suggestions.)
2. Explain why you are going to be writing dialectical journals (see the Appendix) and tell the students you will share one that you wrote on the first chapter.
3. Have the students look at the passage in the chapter that you found particularly interesting and chose to comment on.
4. Read your comment aloud, and invite students to react to both your reference and your comment.
5. Give students a handout showing how you have set out the reference on the left-hand side of the page and the comment on the right (see the Appendix).
6. Ask students to skim through the first chapter and pick out references that they would like to comment on.
7. Have students write their own dialectical journal entry in class as you go around and confirm that they are on the right track.
8. Ask students to share their journal entries in small groups and have them choose one from the group to share with the class.
9. Facilitate a whole-class sharing to show the varied reactions that students have to the text.
10. Set up a reading schedule for the novel and instruct students to come to class with their dialectical journals on the assigned days.

Caveats and Options

1. Have some students select a reference to share with other students who will write a comment on the same reference.
2. Ask students to share their journals in small groups, discuss them, and then share with the rest of the class the entry that caused the most discussion or a question that they would like the rest of the class to consider.
3. Invite students to write an entry on another student's journal entry. This could be organized as a write-and-pass exercise in which students and the instructor sit in a circle, pass around their journals, and write a reaction in every journal they read.
4. Encourage whole-class discussion on a chapter by inviting the sharing of journal entries in the order in which the references appear in the text.
5. As students reach the end of the book, ask them to reread all of their entries before brainstorming together on possible questions for an essay on the text.

References and Further Reading

Achebe, C. (1959). *Things fall apart*. New York: Fawcett Crest.
Alvarez, J. (1991). *How the Garcia girls lost their accents*. New York: Plume.
Anaya, R. (1972). *Bless me, Ultima*. Berkeley, CA: Tonatiuh International.
Kadohata, C. (1989). *The floating world*. New York: Ballantine Books.
Wakatsuki Houston, J., & Houston, J. D. (1974). *Farewell to Manzanar*. New York: Bantam Books.

Appendix

Sample Dialectical Journal Entry Presented to Students

While we are reading our novel, I want you to keep a dialectical journal. The purpose of a dialectical journal is to learn to discover the meaning that a piece of writing has for you. We all respond to a writer's message in a different way, and I would like you to begin to question and investigate how what you read connects with your own views and experiences of life. Below you will find an example of a journal entry that I made on the text.

The Floating World

Reference	Comment
Page 2 The Floating World was the gas station attendants, restaurants, and jobs we depended on, the motel towns floating in the middle of fields and mountains. In old Japan, *ukiyo* meant the districts full of brothels, teahouses, and public baths, but it also referred to change and the pleasures and loneliness change brings. For a long time, I never exactly thought of us as part of any of that. *We* were stable, traveling through an unstable world while my father looked for jobs.	I could imagine nothing worse than living the sort of existence that this family endured. The uncertainty and lack of stability would, I think, drive me crazy. Olivia does not seem to see it like this. She considers the family to be stable and the world to be floating. This is exactly the reverse of how most people would see the situation. I wonder if she means that the family as a unit is so secure that it has created its own sense of permanence. If so, I would, though, expect the relationships between the family members to be particularly close. This doesn't seem to be the case. Look at the relationship between Olivia and Obasan. At times it seems openly hostile, though I get the impression that Obasan does not like to reveal her true feelings. Anyway, I am interested in finding out how the family copes with this Floating World. To me it would be a horrible way of life.

Contributor

Linda Sarmecanic is a Lecturer in the Department of Linguistics and Language Development at San Jose State University, California, in the United States. She has taught English and ESL in England and Iran.

Just Picture It

Levels
Intermediate +

Aims
Enhance reading comprehension

Class Time
1-3 hours

Preparation Time
15-30 minutes

Resources
Literature text

Research has shown that students who are able to visualize as they read perform better on measures of comprehension. Activities such as this one, which encourages learners to picture scenes in their minds as they read, can help form habits that may make learners more effective readers.

Procedure

1. Divide students into groups of three or four. Give each a slip of paper indicating a different descriptive passage from a text the class is currently reading. Ask them not to show the paper to anyone but to read the passage, visualize it in their minds, and draw the scene they see.
2. When everyone is finished, have each group member show the picture to the others, who try to guess which scene from the book it represents.

Caveats and Options

1. To save time, assign the drawings as homework.
2. For lower level or underprepared groups, make guessing easier by providing a list of the various passages that have been assigned, perhaps with one or two extras thrown in as distractors.
3. For extra communicative practice, have pairs of students work together on one picture, with one making suggestions about what to include while the other does the actual drawing.
4. It is very important for the students to realize that to do this task well, they do not have to be good artists. The point is to visualize clearly, then find some way to represent what they see so that it can be recognized.

References and Further Reading

Hodes, C. (1994). Processing visual information: Implications of the dual code theory. *Journal of Instructional Psychology, 21,* 36–43.

Levin, J. (1973). Inducing comprehension in poor readers: A test of a recent model. *Journal of Educational Psychology, 65,* 19–24.

Williams, L. (1983). *Teaching for the two-sided mind.* New York: Simon & Schuster.

Contributor

Claudia Gellert Schulte teaches high school ESOL in Philadelphia, Pennsylvania, in the United States. She holds a master's degree in TESOL from Temple University and is currently working on her doctorate there.

Who Did What When?

Levels
Low intermediate +

Aims
Check understanding of a story line
Develop paraphrasing and retelling skills

Class Time
45-60 minutes

Preparation Time
20 minutes

Resources
Short stories
Plays
Chapters of novels

Caveats and Options

After working together to establish a shared literal understanding of a piece of literature, students are better prepared to engage in more in-depth analysis of the text.

Procedure

1. Write a simplified version of the story line of a text that has been assigned. (See Appendix A and Appendix B for examples.) Write it so that the events are out of sequence.
2. Put students in groups of three or four.
3. Give each group the scrambled story line.
4. Have students number the events according to when they happened in the text.
5. Have students support their answers by locating the events in the text.
6. Have students practice retelling the story line within their groups.
7. Make sure all groups agree on the order of events.
8. For homework, ask the students to read the text again.

1. Vary the complexity of the sentences according to the students' levels.
2. Insert false information into the story line for the students to weed out.
3. Ask students to discard any events that are not essential to the story.
4. Vary the presentation by using strip-story or picture-story formats.
5. If using a picture story, ask the students to write the description for each frame.

References and Further Reading

Collie, J., & Slater, S. (1992). *Literature in the language classroom.* Cambridge: Cambridge University Press.

Duff, A., & Maley, A., (1991). *Literature.* Oxford: Oxford University Press.

Hawthorne, N. (1967). The ambitious guest. In N. Hawthorne, *Selected tales and sketches.* New York: Holt, Rinehart & Winston. (Original work published 1851)

Poe, E. A. (1976). The cask of Amontillado. In S. Levine & S. Levine (Eds.), *The short fiction of Edgar Allan Poe.* Indianapolis, IN: Bobbs-Merrill. (Original work published 1846)

Appendix A: Scrambled Story Line for "The Cask of Amontillado" (Poe, 1846/1976)

Directions: Number the events below according to when they happened in the story.

____ The narrator finishes building the wall.

____ Fortunato insists on going to taste the wine.

____ The narrator vows revenge on Fortunato.

____ He replies "Ugh, ugh, ugh, ugh, ugh, ugh, ugh—it's nothing."

____ The narrator puts Fortunato in chains.

____ The narrator says he has bought a cask of Amontillado and wants Luchesi to judge it.

____ The narrator says that no one has disturbed the wall in 50 years.

__1__ The narrator was insulted by Fortunato.

____ The narrator asks Fortunato about his cough.

____ The narrator runs into Fortunato at the carnival festivities.

____ Fortunato asks the narrator why he is looking for Luchesi.

____ Fortunato screams.

____ The narrator gives Fortunato some wine.

____ The narrator tells Fortunato he is looking for Luchesi.

____ The narrator begins to build a wall in order to trap Fortunato.

____ The narrator leads Fortunato through the catacombs.

Appendix B: Scrambled Picture Story for "The Ambitious Guest" (Hawthorne, 1851/1967)

Cut up the picture story and ask students to put the pictures in order. Then have students practice retelling the story to each other.

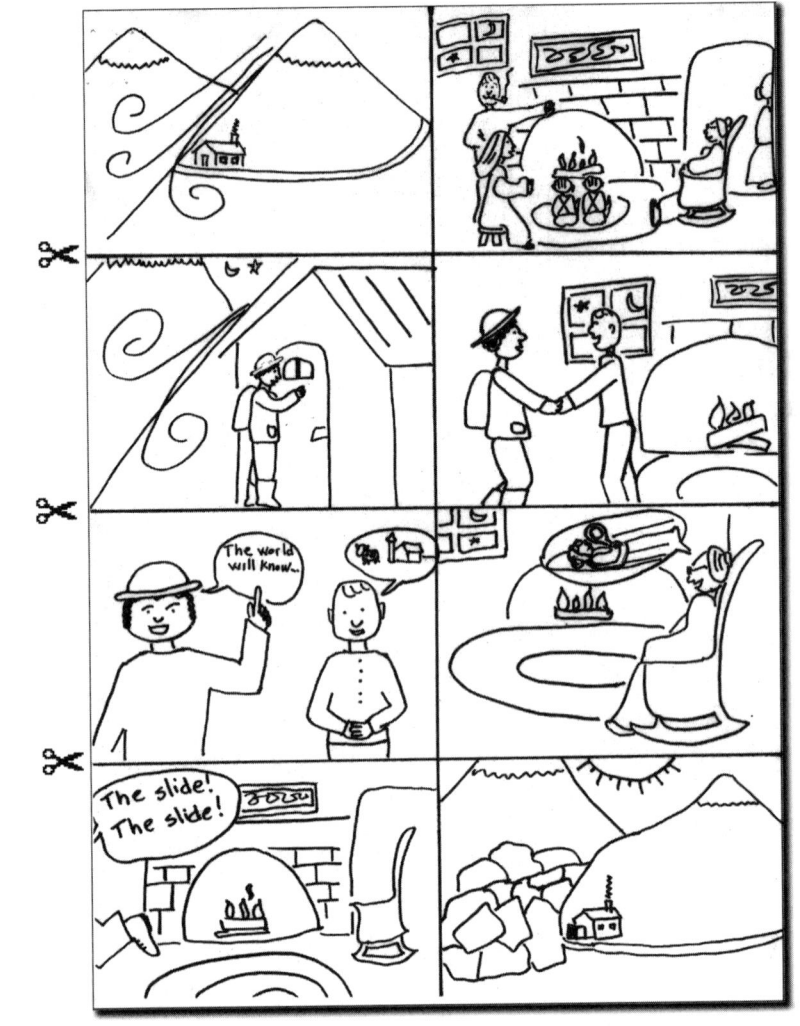

Contributor

Judy Sharkey teaches at Kansai Gaidai College in Japan. She has taught in the Middle East, Latin America, and the United States.

Finding a Description in a Short Story

Levels
Advanced;
heterogeneous
population of young
adults +

Aims
Find aesthetic values in
a literary work
Describe aesthetic
values in literary
characters
Find equivalent values
among people students
know

Class Time
1½ hours

Preparation Time
1½ hours

Resources
Copies of *The Open Boat*, divided into chapters
Facts on Stephen Crane's life and work

A well-chosen literary extract (or a full short story) provides good topics for a variety of activities in the EFL classroom. Description is used in this activity because it is not only a frequently used linguistic phenomenon but also a good means of evaluating human characters.

Procedure

Before the Lesson

1. Divide students into three groups.
2. Give the groups photocopies of *The Open Boat* (Crane, 1897/1993).
   Group 1 gets chapters 1 and 2,
   Group 2 gets chapters 3 and 4,
   Group 3 gets chapters 5 and 6. Do not hand out chapter 7.
3. Ask the students to read the chapters at home.

In Class

1. Give the students cards containing the diagram in Appendix A. Ask the students to ask you questions about the life and work of Stephen Crane to fill in the diagram. Ask one of the students to summarize Crane's life story.
2. Divide students into their original groups.
3. Write the names of the four characters in the story on the chalkboard: the oiler, the cook, the correspondent, the captain. Ask the groups to write a list of characteristics of each of them.
4. Call one member of each group to the chalkboard to write the group's characteristics under each name.

5. Remind the students about the structure of a description:
   - verbs in the present tense
   - the use of appropriate linking words
   - sequencing in order to cover appearance, manner, roles, and relations.
6. Ask four students each to describe one character.
7. Ask students their opinions of the characters (see Appendix B).
8. Ask students what they think the end of the short story is.
9. Give the students the last chapter of the short story (chapter 7) and ask them to read it at home.
10. Assign comprehension questions, true-false statements, topic sentences, scrambled paragraphs, jigsaw reading, and other activities.

Caveats and Options

1. Besides the description of people, deal with the description of nature and places.
2. Ask students to write a paper on an event from their own lives that is similar to an event in the story, bring it to the class, and tell it to their classmates.
3. Ask students to find a writer from their native literary heritage who has written a short story or a novel about a similar topic.
4. Deal with the language of the dialogues in the novel: the differences between speakers or between formal English and colloquial expressions.

References and Further Reading

Collie, J., & Slater, S. (1992). *Literature in the language classroom*. Cambridge: Cambridge University Press.

Crane, S. (1993). *The open boat and other stories*. New York: Dover. (Original work published 1897)

Duff, A., & Maley, A. (1990). *Literature*. Oxford: Oxford University Press.

Hill, J. (1986). *Using literature in language teaching*. New York: Macmillan.

Appendix A: Diagram and Script for Warm-up Activity

DATE	WHAT HAPPENED
1871	
1878	
1883	
Education	
1891–1893	
1893	
1895	
1896–1897	
Jan 2, 1897	
Summer 1897	
1900	

Teacher's Script:

    Stephen Crane was born November 1, 1871. He entered school at the age of seven (1878). In 1883 his family settled in the coastal resort town of Asbury Park, New Jersey.

    Crane never took to schooling. At Syracuse University he distinguished himself as a baseball player but was unable to accept the routine academic life, and after one semester left with no intention of returning.

    In the years 1891–1893 he wrote for newspapers. In 1893 he published his first piece, "An Experiment in Misery."

    In 1895 he published *The Red Badge of Courage*, a document on the American Civil War.

    In 1896–1897 he left New York to cover the insurrection against Spain in Cuba. On January 2, 1897 Crane's ship, *Commodore,* sank off the coast of Florida. He promptly wrote about the this event in "The Open Boat."

    In summer 1897 Crane covered the Greco-Turkish War and later settled in England. He died in Germany on June 5, 1900.

What do you think of the characters?

Appendix B: Questions About the Characters

Do you think their behavior was appropriate?

What do you think about the importance of the brotherhood of man?

How do you value people who do not hesitate to help others when in need?

How would you behave in a similar situation?

Can you give an example of some similar event you have experienced in your life?

Contributor

Eva Tandlichová is Associate Professor and EFL Teacher Trainer at the Department of English and American Studies, Comenius University, Bratislava, Slovakia, and an EFL textbook writer and lecturer.

Quote/Unquote

Levels
Intermediate +

Aims
Be exposed to a wide variety of literature in a short, accessible form

Class Time
2-10 minutes

Preparation Time
5-10 minutes (after initial investment of 2-3 hours)

Resources
Published collections of quotations

By reading and discussing short quotations by a variety of good writers, students are exposed to good literature and learn that it can be directly relevant to their lives. Because the activity includes works by many writers with little expenditure of class time, students become familiar with writers of various cultural backgrounds, women as well as men. Students see that much meaning can be packed into a pithy sentence or two. They gain vocabulary and practice reading and analyzing literature.

Procedure

1. Write a one- to two-sentence quotation on the chalkboard before class begins every day, with the author's name below. (See Appendix for examples.)
2. Explain difficult words and answer vocabulary questions.
3. Ask for possible interpretations.
4. Discuss the quotation briefly. Give brief background information on the author.
5. Ask students to copy the quotation into a designated section of their notebooks, with notes, and to keep all quotations and notes together all semester.

Caveats and Options

1. Find, buy, or borrow from a library at least two collections of quotations (see References and Further Reading); watch for meaningful quotations in the course of your usual reading and copy them into your own special notebook or file for later use in class.
2. Choose quotations with a clear point that is relevant and perhaps inspiring to students.

3. Be inclusive. Seek out quotations from authors of various backgrounds.
4. After doing quotations for several weeks (perhaps halfway through the semester), assign each student a day on which that student will write a quotation of choice on the chalkboard, explain vocabulary, and lead a brief class discussion, just as you have done. Allow students at least a week to find their quotations and give them suggestions about places to find quotations.

References and Further Reading

Bartlett, J., & Kaplan, J. (Eds.). (1992) *Familiar quotations* (16th ed.). Boston: Little, Brown.

Carruth, G., & Ehrlich, E. H. (Eds.). (1988). *The Harper book of American quotations*. New York: Harper & Row.

The concise Oxford dictionary of quotations. (1981). New York: Oxford University Press.

Macmillan dictionary of quotations. (1989). New York: Macmillan.

Partnow, E. (Ed.). (1977). *The quotable woman*. Los Angeles: Pinnacle.

Quotable woman: A collection of shared thoughts. (1989). Philadelphia, PA: Running Press. (Unpaginated)

Tripp, R. (Ed.). (1970). *The international thesaurus of quotations*. New York: Crowell.

Appendix

Examples of quotations that have sparked student interest and discussion:

"Time is the thief you cannot banish." (Phyllis McGinley; in Partnow, 1977, p. 75)

"Justice can never be done in the midst of injustice." (Simone de Beauvoir; in Partnow, 1977, p. 122)

"Only connect." (E. M. Forster; in *Concise Oxford,* 1981, p. 101)

"Think wrongly, if you please, but in all cases think for yourself." (Doris Lessing; in *Quotable Woman,* 1989)

Contributor

"Love from one being to another can only be that two solitudes come nearer, recognize and protect and comfort each other." (Han Suyin; in Partnow, 1977, p. 220)

"You may be disappointed if you fail, but you are doomed if you don't try." (Beverly Sills; in *Quotable Woman,* 1989)

Stephanie Vandrick is Assistant Professor in the ESL Department, University of San Francisco, California, in the United States. She also teaches Women's Studies courses and writes about sociopolitical issues and literature.

Multicultural Ideas

Levels
Intermediate +

Aims
Read novels and short stories in English

Class Time
Variable

Preparation Time
Variable

Resources
Novels and short stories by authors who share the students' cultural background

Caveats and Options

By reading books that allow them to concentrate on the story development for which they possess the schema, students are less frustrated than when they have to try to understand both the language and the culture.

Procedure

1. If you have a homogeneous class, choose a story or novel that is written about the country or culture that they share.
2. If you have a heterogeneous class, find an appropriate text for each student.
3. Explain to the students that you want them to keep a dialectical journal in which they write their reactions to what they are required to read. Tell them that you do not want a summary, only their opinions. If necessary, share something you have written about a book you read. Explain that they are reading for pleasure; they do not need to understand every word.

1. This activity is an opportunity to stretch the students intellectually. Once they get over the idea that they need to understand everything, they will begin to enjoy reading.
2. Allow some leeway; Asians will probably understand other Asian writers (even if they are writing about another Asian country) better than they will understand a story set in Africa.
3. See Appendix for a list of some excellent authors who write about the cultures they know and understand.

Appendix: List of Authors

Amy Tan, Timothy Mo, Gish Gen, Fae Myenne Ng, Liu Sola (China)
Sandra Cisneros, Rudolfo A. Anaya (Hispanic in the U.S.)
Chinua Achebe, Ben Okri, Wole Soyinka, Ama Ata Aidoo (Africa)
Kamala Markandaya, Bharati Mukherjee, V.S. Naipaul, Salman Rushdie, Hanif Kureishi, Rohinton Mistry, Shashi Deshpande (India)
Jamaica Kinkaid, Derek Walcott, George Lamming, Caryl Phillips (Caribbean)
Kazuo Ishiguro, John Okada, Pico Iyer (Japan)
Catherine Lim, Edwin Thumboo (Singapore)
William Olen Butler (Vietnam)
Witi Ihimaera (Maori)
Romesh Gunesekara, Michael Ondaatje (Sri Lanka)
Laura Esquivel (Mexico)
Isabel Allende, Gabriel García Marquez, Jorge Luis Borges, Carlos Fuentes, Mario Vargas Llosa, Octavio Paz (South America)
Nejib Mafouz (Egypt)
Han Su Yin, K.S. Maniam (Chinese Malaysia)
Sembene Ousmane (Senegal)

Contributor

Valerie Whiteson, English and ESL Instructor at Evergreen Valley College, San Jose, California, is coauthor of Personal Themes in Literature: The Multicultural Experience *(Prentice-Hall Regents, 1993).*

All-Purpose Dialogue Journal Preview Questions

Levels
High intermediate +;
secondary +

Aims
Use ideas about and responses to stories as topics for dialogue journals

Class Time
About 15 minutes at the beginning of the course

Preparation Time
1-3 hours

Resources
Short story anthologies or course textbook

Giving students prompts for journals provides a guide for the kind of writing and topics you expect and expands their ways to explore a story. When students have the questions ahead of time, they can choose to read the story with the questions in mind. Having the same questions for all the stories encourages comparison and contrast across stories.

Procedure

1. Explain to students that dialogue journals are a way to make sure they understand the story and to explore their reactions—not simply to summarize. Tell them that you will not mark errors but will respond with requests for clarification and comments.
2. Give students specific questions for each story (see the Appendix). However, for any story, tell students that they may also choose an additional topic from among the given list, as appropriate.

Caveats and Options

1. Have students write a detailed response to just one question or shorter answers to several; have them write about something else.

References and Further Reading

Peyton, J. K. (Ed.). (1990). *Students and teachers writing together: Perspectives on journal writing.* Alexandria, VA: TESOL.

Spack, R. (1994). *The international story: An anthology with guidelines for reading and writing about fiction.* New York: St. Martin's Press.

Appendix: List of Questions

1. What words didn't you know? Write them and put your best guess at the meaning, for example, "some type of animal."
2. What is the overall emotion/mood of the story? How does the author create this mood—with what details?
3. What emotion do you think a particular character is feeling? How do you know?
4. What is the message or moral of the story? Do you agree?
5. How does a particular character's attitude toward something compare to your own attitude?
6. Did you find a confusing passage in the story? Which part do you not understand? What do you think it means?
7. How does the author use examples to support a point?
8. If you were to create a filmed advertisement (a "preview") for a movie based on this story, which two scenes would you select? Why?
9. Give advice to one of the characters.
10. Which character do you sympathize with most? Why?
11. What choices did a particular character face? Why did she make those particular choices? What do you think about her choices, and the consequences?
12. Looking back at the whole story, can you say what, precisely, was the point at which the outcome became inevitable? Why do you think this? If you do not think there was such a point, give your reasons for thinking that the outcome was not inevitable.
13. Each event in a story is tied to what happens before it and will in turn affect what happens afterwards. List several important events in the story. For each one, briefly summarize (a) what happened before this that caused or connects to it, and (b) what happens after this, as a result or consequence.
14. Write a brief account of this story from one of the character's point of view.
15. Using clues from the story, determine the approximate age of one of the characters. What do you know about people of that age that might help you understand this story?
16. Examine the images and words in the story. Do any words or phrases appeal to your sense of sight? sound? taste? smell? touch? Does one

type predominate? Do any of these relate to a character's moral or emotional state?

17. Analyze one character in the story. Describe this person's outward appearance and behavior. What are his inner emotional and moral qualities? Include positive and negative characteristics; most important values; conflicts being experienced (external and internal), choices being faced, and changes happening (if any).

18. Assume that a local newspaper has found out about what the characters did and assigns you the task of covering the story. Write a newspaper article describing the incident, including quotations from the story—perhaps in the form of interviews with the characters. Divide into three groups to write three different styles of article: (a) for a newspaper that sensationalizes its stories; (b) for a newspaper that gives the personal "human" angle of a story; and (c) for a newspaper that provides straightforward coverage of its stories. Be sure to provide a headline for the article.

Contributor

Lise Winer teaches in the TESOL and Applied Linguistics programs at Southern Illinois University, Carbondale, Illinois, in the United States.

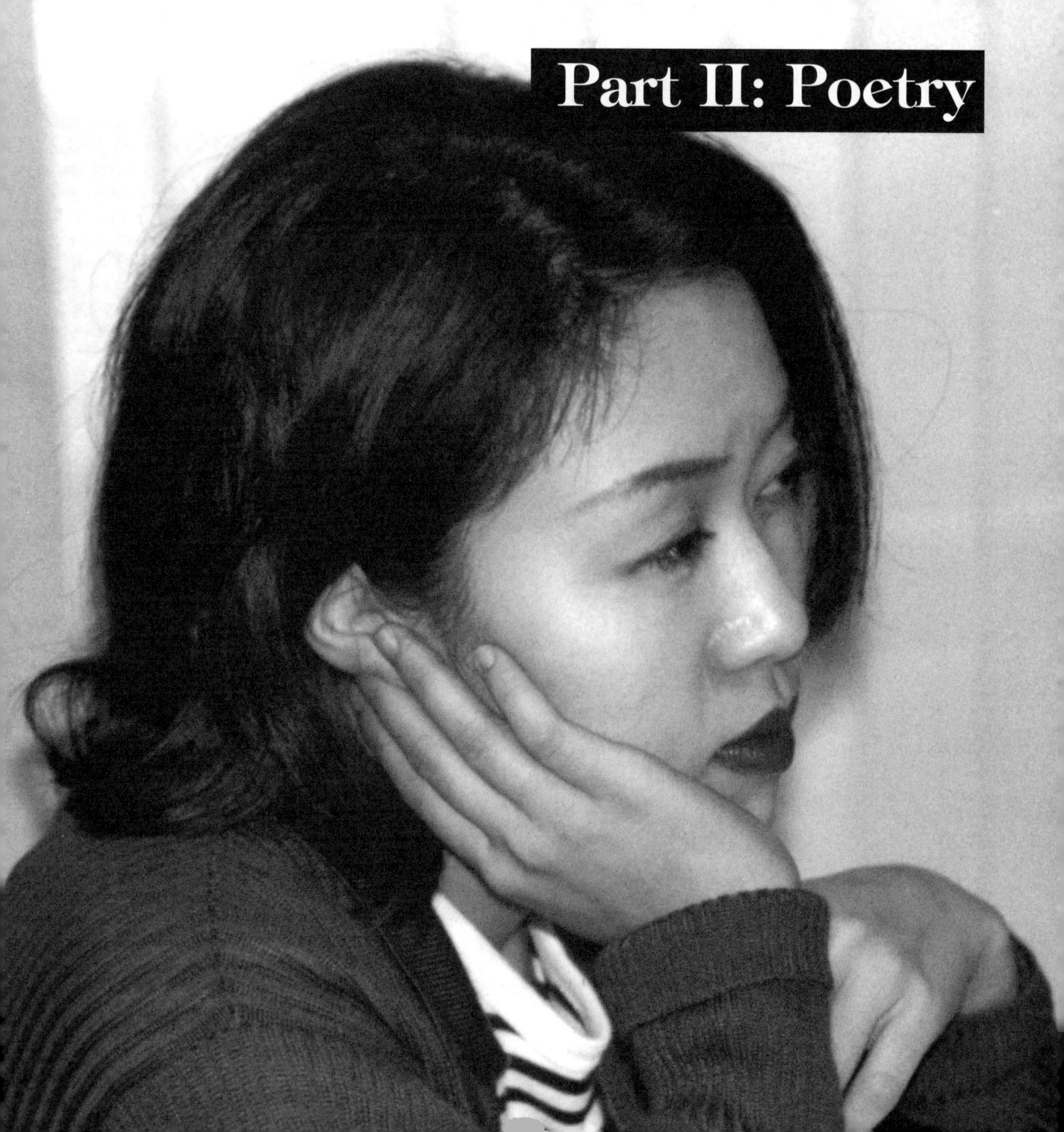

Part II: Poetry

Jee Hae Kwon at Eurocentres, Alexandria, Virginia USA.

Introduction

If you have never taught poetry in your ESOL classroom, you will be surprised and gratified by the students' enjoyment of the poems you love. There are teachers who even talk about "the joy of teaching poetry." Choosing poems that work is not easy; but once you have found one, it will probably work with other groups. Many students are flattered when you teach them a poem by a famous poet. Don't underestimate the intelligence of a class; students are challenged by a poem that is somewhat difficult. After I explain "My Last Duchess," by Robert Browning, for instance, students usually ask for more poems like that.

There are many reasons why studying poetry, and even writing poetry, improve sentence structure and help students to focus on vocabulary, rhythm, stress, and the use of metaphor and similes. Above all, poets use language in fresh and exciting ways. Most of our students are afraid to be adventurous when expressing themselves.

By reading the ideas of the writers in this section and trying some of them out, you will most certainly come up with original and different ways of introducing poetry in your classes.

Out of respect to copyright, we have not included the texts of poems. After checking your own and other libraries for the poems, however, you might try finding them on the Internet. One possible World Wide Web site for the poems of Emily Dickinson is:
    http://www.cc.columbia.edu/acis/bartleby/dickinson/ed100.htm
Another useful address is:
    http://www.ling.lancs.ac.uk/visitors/kenji/literatu.htm

Using Borrowed Lines

Levels
Intermediate +;
secondary +

Aims
Focus on a writer's
imagery
Be creative with English
without worrying about
correctness

Class Time
Variable

Preparation Time
30 minutes

Resources
Short story or novel that
the students are reading

When students are reading a story, their first order of business is generally to understand the basics, the who-what-where. When you want them to linger over a passage, to reread and savor the author's words, you can ask them to create a poem based on the passage.

Procedure

1. Have students look at a familiar excerpt from a story or novel. Ask them to read aloud words, phrases, or sentences that appeal to them, ones that create images in their minds.
2. Show them a short poem or poems that you have created by borrowing lines you like. For example, here is a poem created about a character in *The House on Mango Street,* by Sandra Cisneros (1991). The author borrowed phrases from "Louie, His Cousin & His Other Cousin" and "Marin":

MARIN
in the doorway
clicking her fingers
looks at boys and is not afraid
dancing, singing
under the streetlight
waiting for someone to change her life

3. Turn to the reading the students are currently doing (another story or novel, or another passage from the same one). Ask the students to create borrowed poems of their own. Ask them to focus on a particular character, setting, incident, or idea from the reading. Students should also choose titles for their poems.

4. When you return to class, students can share their borrowed poems by
    - writing them on the board
    - posting them on the walls
    - circulating them via networked computers.

Caveats and Options

1. Writing is best done out of class, with 20 to 30 minutes spent in class for sharing the results.
2. Students who wish to write original poems should be free to do so. Ask them to maintain the focus on some aspect of the story, novel, passage under discussion. Students can also begin with an image from the text and then write their own poem.

References and Further Reading

Cisneros, S. (1991). *The house on Mango Street.* New York: Vintage Contemporaries.

Contributor

Linda Butler teaches ESL, writes, and consults in Massachusetts, in the United States. She is the creator of The ESOL Reader's Companion *series published by McGraw-Hill.*

Poem Charades

Levels
Any

Aims
Become interested in reading and writing
Increase vocabulary

Class Time
20-40 minutes

Preparation Time
10 minutes

Resources
Poems

This cooperative task promotes students' interest in reading and writing by encouraging creative expression and active interpretation. Through poetic communication, students can associate words with vivid imagery.

Procedure

1. Divide the class into an even number of groups, calling each group either an A or a B group.
2. Hand out a simple poem to the A groups and a different poem to the B groups. Ask the students to read the poem.
3. Have students in each group briefly discuss the basic meaning of the poem.
4. Model the acting out of a sample poem in a lively manner.
5. Have the A groups act out the action of their poem for the B groups after preparing, and vice versa.
6. Have each group write a poem to match the action they saw in the other group's performance.
7. Have A and B groups exchange the original poems and compare their own version with the original.
8. Discuss the poems as a class.

Caveats and Options

1. If students are shy or the poem is difficult, substitute drawing for acting.
2. Tell students that it is fine if their version and the original poem differ.
3. Short action- or emotion-oriented poems, such as nursery rhymes and song lyrics, make excellent materials.

Contributor

David George is a Lecturer at Kansai Gaidai College, Hirakata City, Osaka, Japan.

Poetic Slips

Levels
Any

Aims
Explore the cohesive devices used in poetry

Class Time
Variable

Preparation Time
10 minutes

Resources
Poem written line by line on slips of paper
Basket

Dissecting a poem and having the students reassemble it draws attention to the tools of poetry—rhythm, rhyme, and imagery. The process enhances students' understanding of why the poet used words in a particular way.

Procedure

1. Place the slips of paper into the basket.
2. Arrange the seats in a circle. Have the students sit down, take a slip of paper from the basket, and read their line of poetry silently.
3. Read the first line of the poem aloud. Have the student who thinks he or she has the next line read out the line. Continue until all the lines have been read out and the poem has been reassembled.
4. When arguments arise about the line order, examine what the poet wrote, look at the written clues, and explore possible reasons for a particular order.

Caveats and Options

1. The difficulty of this activity will vary with the complexity of the poem being studied. (Use easier poems with beginners and more obscure ones with advanced students.)
2. Focus on a particular aspect of language. For example, to draw the students' attention to the adjectives used, distribute only adjectives to half of the class (Group A) and the lines with their adjectives missing to the other students (Group B). Follow the steps above, except that when a student from Group B reads out his line, have somebody from Group A supply an appropriate adjective.
3. If students have studied a poem previously, distribute phrases rather than full lines. This activity then acts as a reinforcement of or a check on the students' understanding.

4. With longer poems, divide the class into groups and give each group lines from a verse. First, within the group, have members order their lines to form a verse as described earlier. Then have the groups order the verses to form the poem. If appropriate, have half of the group act out the verse while the other half recites it.

Contributor

Geraldine Hetherton is an EFL Lecturer at Fukui Prefectural University, Japan, and has also taught in Europe, Africa, and the Middle East.

The Numbers Game: 5-7-5

Levels
Any

Aims
Write creative summaries of long texts

Class Time
20-30 minutes

Preparation Time
5 minutes

Resources
Original text

Haiku are relatively easy and enjoyable to write and can provide a concise, memorable summary of a short story, novel, or play.

Procedure

1. Have students study the selected text (see References and Further Reading).
2. Explain the fundamentals of writing a haiku: three lines with five, seven, and five syllables per line, respectively.
3. Ask the students to write a haiku about one of the following:
   - their overall impression of the text
   - a character
   - the climax of the scene
   - a summary of the action

   Or divide the class into groups and assign one of the above topics to each group. Read some samples of haiku aloud.
4. Decide on a pleasing order for the recitation of the haiku. An effective way is to set up a round in which haiku types are recited in a particular order and that order (e.g., summary, impression, character(s), climax) is repeated until all students have performed their piece. Have the students use voice techniques to build to a climatic finish.

Caveats and Options

1. Choose a text to suit the language ability of your students, demand higher standards of sophistication from your more able students, or both.
2. Have the students rewrite an act, or indeed a whole play, in haiku by assigning one scene to each group and asking them to write a haiku

for that scene. Then divide each group in half, with one half acting and the other reciting in a performance of the act or play.
3. Limericks are an equally useful medium for this activity.

References and Further Reading

Friel, B. (1994). *Molly Sweeney*. Dublin, Ireland: Gallery Press.

Appendix: Haiku Based on the Character Molly Sweeney (Friel, 1994)

Molly Sweeney

I long know the dark.	5
Why change everything with light?	7
But hear his urgings.	5

Contributor

Geraldine Hetherton is an EFL Lecturer at Fukui Prefectural University, Japan, and has also taught in Europe, Africa, and the Middle East.

Rhyme Time

Levels
Intermediate +

Aims
Think and write creatively
Recognize phonetic similarities between words

Class Time
Variable

Resources
Samples of short rhyming verse (preferably light humor)
Rhyming worksheet

Procedure

1. Have students take turns reading aloud short rhyming verse, such as that of Ogden Nash (see References and Further Reading).
2. Discuss why the verse is or isn't interesting or humorous.
3. Have students work on the rhyming worksheet (see Appendix) either individually, in pairs, or in groups.
4. Have students develop other rhyming word possibilities.
5. Show them the rhyming sequences in four-stanza poems: AABB, ABAB, —A—A. Explain that each line should be similar in length.
6. Have them write rhyming poems (four lines or more) on a topic of their choice in pairs or in small groups.
7. Share and discuss the students' poems in class.

Caveats and Options

1. Assist any student having trouble. Writing even simple poems can be difficult for many people.
2. If some students are nervous about reading their own poems in class, read the poems anonymously.
3. Use this activity as a springboard for a more serious look at writing and enjoying poetry.
4. Do the rhyming worksheet orally in the form of a game with groups competing to find the most rhymes for particular words. You may not need to hand out the worksheet.

References and Further Reading

Harmon, W. (Ed.). (1979). *The Oxford book of American light verse*. New York: Oxford University Press.

Appendix: Rhyme Time Worksheet

How many words can you think of that rhyme with:

pen　　　*red*　　　*feet*　　　*sing*　　　*cake*　　　*hat*

men

hen

den

ten

then

when

Can you make other rhyming lists?

(a) _____　　(b) _____　　(c) _____　　(d) _____　　(e) _____

1.

2.

3.

4.

5.

6.

You can use the above lists to help you in writing your poems.

Contributor

Richard Humphries is a Lecturer at Kansai Gaidai College, Hirakata City, Japan.

Act It Out

Levels
Intermediate +

Aims
Read a narrative poem with enjoyment
Improve comprehension and composition skills

Class Time
Variable

Preparation Time
15 minutes

Resources
Narrative poem

Caveats and Options

References and Further Reading

Contributor

Most students agree that poetry is the most challenging genre in literature. By rewriting a poem in a script and acting it out, students can appreciate and understand poetry better.

Procedure

1. Have students read a narrative poem with an interesting plot (see References and Further Reading).
2. Hand out an example of a script. If possible, show them an example of a narrative poem for which the script is written.
3. If the poem consists of many plots, choose a plot or scene.
4. Divide the students into groups according to the number of roles in the plot or scene.
5. Have students rewrite the scene in a script for a play. Encourage them to make the language more lively and realistic.
6. Act out the play.

1. Encourage creativity and imagination.
2. Do not choose a scene that is more than two pages long.

Poems that work well include Robert Browning's "My Last Duchess," E.A. Robinson's "Mr. Flood's Party," and Percy Bysshe Shelley's "Ozymandias," all of which are widely anthologized.

Anita Lie, English and EFL Instructor in the English Department, Petra Christian University, Surabaya, Indonesia, writes articles for scholarly and popular publications.

Experiencing the Music of Poetry: Poe's "Annabel Lee"

Levels
Intermediate +

Aims
Improve pronunciation, rhythm, and intonation
Read a well-known literary work

Class Time
Variable

Preparation Time
Variable
Resources
Copies of "Annabel Lee"

Poetry reading offers students an enjoyable and stimulating way to improve their pronunciation, rhythm, and intonation.

Procedure

1. If desired, provide students with background information about the poet and the poem:
   - Edgar Allan Poe (1809-1849) was a U.S. writer whose poems are famous for their rhyme and repetition.
   - "Annabel Lee" (Edgar Allan Poe, in Sullivan, 1978) is an account of his wife, Virginia Clemm, who died of tuberculosis.
2. Read the poem aloud to students. Ask them to pay attention to the rhyming and sounds without focusing on the meaning of the words. Special features to note are
   - rhyming: Tell them to listen for the words that rhyme with Lee.
   - repetition: Tell them to listen for the repetition of certain words.
3. Hand out copies of the poem to the students. With the students following the text, read the first stanza of the poem. Review the unknown vocabulary words. Ask the students to identify specific examples of Poe's use of rhyming and repetition within the stanza. Use this approach for the remaining stanzas. (See Appendix A for examples.)
4. Read the poem line by line, having students repeat each line in chorus. Recite the poem along with the students, helping them keep up the beat. As they repeat, students may tap or clap the beat.
5. Discuss the meaning and the mood of the poem.
6. Have individual students read stanzas of the poem aloud.

Caveats and Options

1. Make a recording of this poem for students to listen to in the language lab or at home. Students can practice reading along with this recording.
2. If possible, find a professionally recorded reading of the poem to play for the students.
3. Have students practice reading the poem as homework to recite for the next class period.
4. Ask the students to memorize the poem.
5. Give the students comprehension questions to answer rather than having an open discussion of the poem. (See Appendix B.)
6. Use the poem for vocabulary development. (See Appendix C.)

References and Further Reading

Sullivan, N. (Ed.). (1978). *The treasury of American poetry.* New York: Dorset Press.

Appendix A: Examples of Poe's Use of Rhyming and Repetition

1. Rhyming at the End of Lines

   - In the first four stanzas (26 lines) every other line ends with *sea, Lee,* or *me*.
   - In the fifth stanza the second and third lines end with *we,* which rhymes with the three words given above.
   - In the sixth stanza the first and third lines end with *sea*.
   - In the seventh stanza the second and fourth lines end with *Lee,* and the seventh and eighth lines end with *sea*.
   - Every stanza except the sixth ends with *sea, Lee,* or *me*.

2. Internal Rhyming

   In the last stanza there are three instances of internal rhyming (italics added):

   For the moon never *beams* without bringing me *dreams*
   And the stars never *rise* but I see the bright *eyes*
   And so, all the *nighttide,* I lie down by the *side*

3. Repetition
- The name *Annabel Lee* is mentioned in every stanza except the fifth.
- The following phrases are repeated more than once:

    a kingdom by the sea (5 times)
    of the beautiful Annabel Lee (3 times)

- Some phrases are repeated with only slight variation:

    a wind blew out of a cloud by night (line 15)
    the wind came out of the cloud (line 25)
    chilling my Annabel Lee (line 16)
    chilling and killing my Annabel Lee (lines 25-26)
    And this was the reason (line 13)
    Yes! that was the reason (line 23)
    In her sepulcher there by the sea (line 40)
    in her tomb by the side of the sea (line 41)

- Some words are repeated in the same sentence (italics added):

    It was *many* and *many* a year ago
    She was a *child* and I was a *child*
    But we *loved* with a *love* that was more than *love*
    can ever dissever my *soul* from the *soul*
    Of *my darling*, *my darling*, my life and my bride

Appendix B: Comprehension Questions

1. Where did Annabel Lee live?
2. Who envied Annabel Lee and the poet?
3. Why did she die?
4. Where is Annabel Lee now?
5. Why can no one separate the poet from his beloved Annabel Lee?

Appendix C: Vocabulary Development

Directions: Substitute a word from the list below for the highlighted words in the sentences adapted from the poem.

carried   made cold   desired   were jealous of

1. The winged seraphs *coveted* her and me. _____
2. The angels *envied* her and me. _____
3. Her kinsmen *bore* her away from me. _____
4. The wind *chilled* my Annabel Lee. _____

Directions: Give the proper word forms for each word.

to covet

1. Mr. Jones was _____ of his neighbor's car.

to chill

2. The winter air was _____.

to envy

3. Maria tried to hide her _____ of her friend's success.

to bear

4. The athlete found the pain _____.

Contributors

Christine Meloni, Associate Professor of EFL at The George Washington University, in Washington, DC, in the United States, is the author of several articles and a textbook on developing oral skills and on using literature in the ESOL classroom. Candace Matthews, Assistant Professor of EFL at The George Washington University, is the author of several textbooks focusing on oral communication skills.

What Is a Poem (Not)?

Levels
Intermediate +

Aims
Understand the importance of verbal economy in poetry

Class Time
1 hour

Preparation Time
15–30 minutes

Resources
Copies of a short poem

What makes poetic language poetic? Widdowson (1992) believes that because poems achieve their effects in such elusive ways, the best way to become aware of what affects the reader is to contrast the poem with a variant version of it, in which some of the language has been changed. This activity makes a direct point about verbal economy and requires little prior experience with poetry.

Procedure

1. Choose a short, unrhymed poem, at least slightly ambiguous in meaning, and distribute a copy to each student. The poem should contain some sentence fragments or other incomplete utterances, perhaps some run-on sentences, and few adjectives. Read it aloud and clarify unfamiliar vocabulary items. Have students offer some ideas as to what it is about without paraphrasing it or coming to definite conclusions.
2. Pretend (though not too convincingly) to be shocked that the poem should contain sentence fragments or run-ons and complain that this keeps you from fully understanding what the poet is trying to say. Then express your additional belief that the poem's lack of descriptive adjectives makes it too "plain."
3. Assign students the task of "fixing" the poem by rewriting it in full, completely grammatical sentences. Tell them to make run-ons into separate sentences, each with its own subject. Tell them also to make the poem more "beautiful" by adding lots of descriptive adjectives. They should try to stay as close as possible to the poem's meaning as they understand it.
4. Duplicate some of the results and, with the class, compare them with the original. Ask students whether they think any of the rewritings are

actually improvements, and why or why not. Discuss the value of verbal economy in poetry as well as the differences between poetry and various forms of prose such as journals.

5. If the students have already written poems of their own, have them go back over them to eliminate excess verbiage in the light of what they have learned.

Caveats and Options

1. If you fear some students might take your act too seriously (or if you're not an actor), ask them instead, "How would this poem be rewritten by a person who believed that (a) everyone should write in nothing but completely grammatical sentences and (b) all good writing has to have lots of descriptive adjectives?"
2. Have students rewrite the poems in groups. Aside from benefiting those students who may find the task confusing, it can also lead to interesting negotiations about what meanings the poet may or may not have intended and whether proposed additions might overly distort them.
3. Some students or groups may need a more explicit meaning for the original poem as a basis for completing the task. If you offer one, make sure the students understand that your explanation can never be the same as what the poet really meant but can only point them toward it.
4. Another way of making students aware of the differences between poetry and prose, advocated by Widdowson (1992) and others, is to compare poetic and prose versions of similar subject matter. Widdowson (1992, chapter 8) offers an example from literature.

References and Further Reading

Widdowson, H. G. (1992). *Practical stylistics.* Oxford: Oxford University Press.

Contributor

Claudia Gellert Schulte teaches high school ESOL and is a doctoral student at Temple University in Philadelphia, Pennsylvania, in the United States. Her main interests are vocabulary, poetry, and cognitive processes in second language acquisition.

Note to a Plum Thief

Levels
Intermediate +

Aims
Become familiar with nonrhymed poetic language

Class Time
40 minutes

Preparation Time
10 minutes

Resources
Copies of the poem "This is Just to Say"

One of the major obstacles in getting students to write poetry is that, apart from rhyme, many of them have never thought about what makes a poem different from other forms of writing. One way of giving them a feel for unrhymed poetic language—and convincing them that they can write it—is to have them respond to a "message" poem with a message of their own, written in the form of the original.

Procedure

1. Give each student a copy of "This is Just to Say," by William Carlos Williams (1938/1951). (This poem, written to sound like a note left on a table, apologizes for eating some plums that the recipient of the note was probably saving for breakfast. Each line contains between one and three words.)
2. Ask the class if they think this is really a poem and, if so, what makes it one.
3. At some point, discuss how poems often use short, patterned lines to give shape and rhythm to a message as well as to draw the reader's attention to certain words, images, and meanings.
4. Ask the students to imagine that they have just found this note on their kitchen table and to write a response to it using the same form (just a few words on each line).
5. With the authors' permission, read some of the results out loud.
6. As a follow-up assignment, ask students to think of something they would like to say to someone they know (or someone in the public eye) and to write it out using the same form. Again, read the results out loud.

Caveats and Options

1. Students should feel free to write either a plain, straightforward message or something more whimsical or imaginative. At the same time, be sure they understand that although any content is acceptable here because the point is to learn about form, form in itself is not enough to make something a poem.
2. Widdowson (1992) discusses this poem in terms of how its very ordinariness provokes us into finding "an undercurrent of implied significance in it" (p. 29)—that is, it is a subtle representation of mixed guilt and gratification. Koch (1973) uses this same theme more explicitly to inspire a "poetry idea" for writing: "apologizing for something you're really secretly glad you did" (p. 100). You may want to explore these ideas as well.

References and Further Reading

Dunning, S., Lueders, E., & Smith, H. (Eds.). (1966). *Reflections on a gift of watermelon pickle.* New York: Scholastic Book Services.

Koch, K. (1973). *Rose, where did you get that red? Teaching great poetry to children.* New York: Random House.

Widdowson, H. G. (1992). *Practical stylistics.* Oxford: Oxford University Press.

Williams, W. C. (1951). This is just to say. In *Collected earlier poems.* New York: New Directions. (Original work published 1938)

Contributor

Claudia Gellert Schulte teaches high school ESOL in Philadelphia, Pennsylvania, in the United States. She holds an MA in TESOL from Temple University and is currently working on her doctorate there.

Poetry for Pronunciation, Pronunciation for Poetry

Levels
Low intermediate +;
ages 8 +

Aims
Practice pronunciation of specific consonant and vowel patterns
Practice English intonation and rhythmic patterns
Learn about U.S. and British culture as expressed through poetry

Preparation Time
15-30 minutes

Resources
Anthology of British/U.S. poetry

In this activity, students take advantage of the sounds and natural rhythms of poetry to reinforce English language pronunciation patterns. For older students who may be interested primarily in vocational or technical English, this type of activity may be the only acceptable way (from their point of view) to introduce them to the insights revealed through literature in general and to the richness of U.S. and British poetry in particular. The poetry thus becomes a vehicle for discussing attributes of U.S. language and culture.

Procedure

1. Teach a chosen pronunciation, stress, or intonation pattern.
2. Chose a poem that exemplifies the pronunciation pattern, and direct-teach the vocabulary needed to understand the poem.
3. Discuss some cultural issue or issues that will facilitate comprehension of the poem.
4. Read the poem to the class to model the pronunciation, stress, or intonation pattern that was originally practiced.
5. Reread the poem with the class as a choral reading, or pair the students and have them reread the poem with their partner.
6. Ask the class to identify where the pronunciation, stress, or intonation pattern that was practiced appears in the poem.
7. Divide the class into pairs or small groups and ask them to interpret the poem.
8. Have the groups choose a spokesperson who will report the interpretation back to the class.
9. Discuss the interpretations with the class.

Caveats and Options

1. Avoid lengthy poems. Limit the activity to poems of one page or less.
2. Be sure that the poem exemplifies the pronunciation pattern the class has been practicing. It is well known that U.S. technical students often question the relevance of learning poetry, and many international students share that view. However, if they perceive that the poetry will help their pronunciation, students will afterwards become more open to spending time exploring and discussing the cultural implications of the poetry.
3. I have used this exercise successfully in conjunction with Orion (1988).

References and Further Reading

Hughes, L. (1974). *Selected poems*. New York: Vintage Books.
McMichael, G. (Ed.). (1985). *Concise anthology of American literature* (2nd ed.). New York: Macmillan.
Orion, G. F. (1988). *Pronouncing American English*. New York: Newbury House.

Contributor

Dorothy Solé teaches at Miami-Dade Community College and works in the writing lab of the University of Miami, Florida, in the United States.

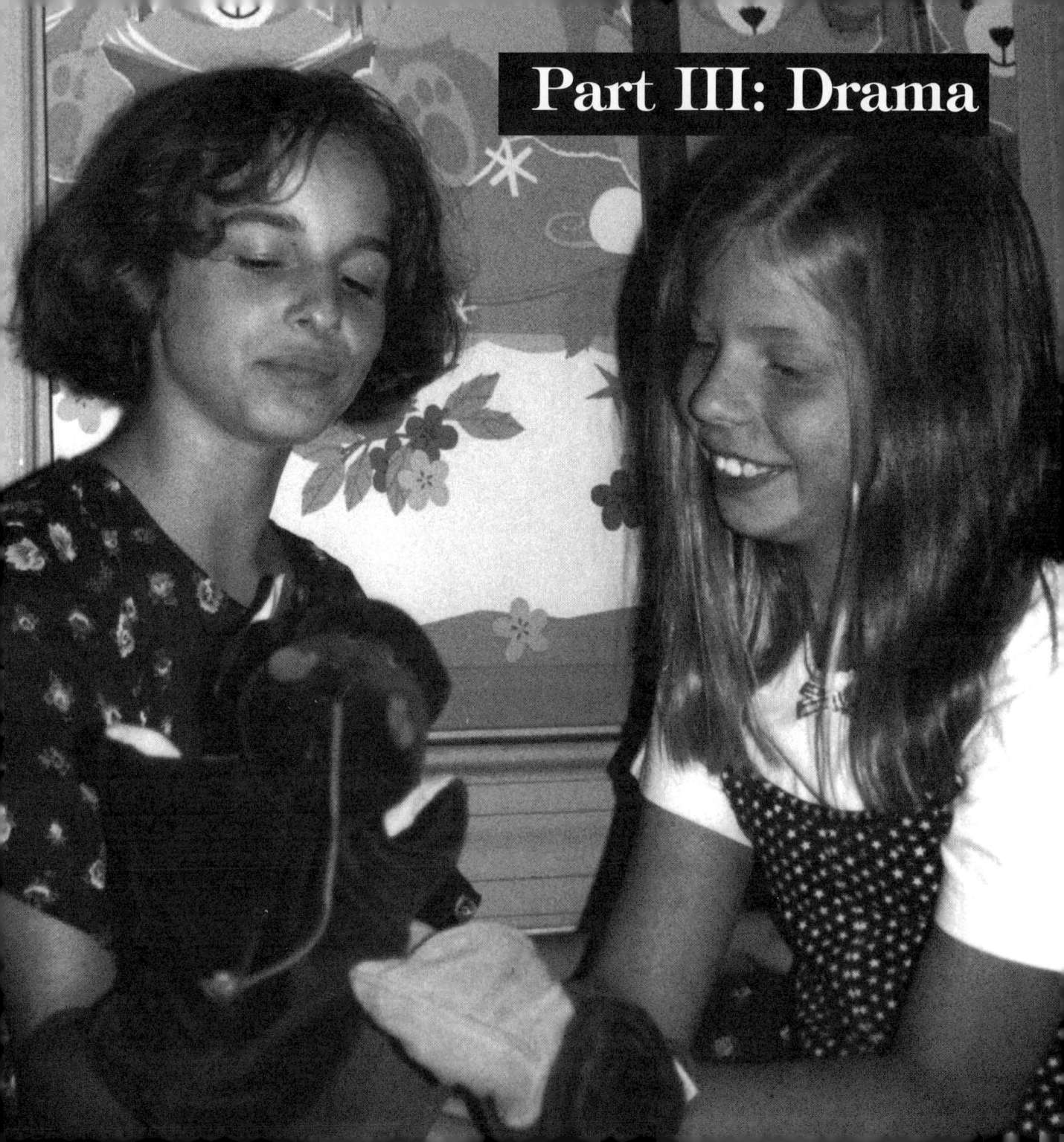

Left to right: Karolina Gendek and Anya Nowakowski, Bethesda, Maryland USA.

Introduction

Drama in the ESOL classroom can be seen from three perspectives: as literature, as public performance, and as improvisation. From the point of view of literature and public performance, drama provides a rich resource for exploring theoretical and practical aspects of language. The improvisation aspect gives students opportunities for developing their communicative competence.

Most plays are rich in dialogue. By using them in the classroom we can focus on conversation in an exciting and useful way. Most good drama needs interpretation. We have to move beyond the surface of the words to make sense of what is being said. By asking our students to do this, we are helping them to understand conversational discourse.

Many teachers who use drama in the classroom try to choose plays that are available in film or video form. By carefully choosing to show the movie either before or after studying the play, these teachers add an invaluable dimension to their students' appreciation of the work. One of the best experiences I have had was to take a class to see Arthur Miller's *Death of a Salesman,* produced by the local repertory theater. They have never forgotten the experience, nor have I.

Contributors to this volume describe exciting and novel ways to use drama in the ESOL classroom. By introducing students to English drama and real literature, we pay them the compliment that they are capable of enjoying the best that English has to offer. Ultimately, we hope, some of these students will develop a love for English that will help to make it truly their second language.

Acting Is Becoming

Levels
High beginning +

Aims
Enhance descriptive language abilities
Develop language and cultural skills through dramatic play
Build self-confidence in experimenting with language

Class Time
30 minutes per step, divided among seven class periods

Preparation Time
Minimal

Resources
Paper
Crayons or markers
Discarded catalogues and magazines

Expanding self-created characters is a wonderful tool for learning language and culture and for enhancing students' self-esteem as learners. Students have a great deal of latitude in deciding who they want to be as speakers of English (or another language) and in trying out new linguistic and cultural behaviors in a nonthreatening way.

Procedure

1. Have students brainstorm several sets of descriptive vocabulary, including words for
   - physical characteristics
   - personality traits
   - occupations and hobbies
   - family members
2. Ask each student to either draw a picture of a character they would like to be, cut out a picture from a magazine, or create a composite picture.
3. Once they have drawn or otherwise created their character, have the students write a description of the character in the first person; for example, "I have red hair and gray eyes. I am married and have three children. I like running and spending time outdoors. I enjoy sewing, painting and music. I am usually happy, but I also have a temper."
4. Have the students share their pictures with each other, as a class if it is small or in groups of two or three students.
5. Create a series of scenarios involving two or three characters, for example, "Person A wants to buy a new bicycle. Person B is trying to convince him to buy a moped, instead. Each person is trying to persuade the other." Ask the students to respond to the scenarios as their characters would.

6. Have students write their own scenarios in groups of two or three, incorporating their characters into the scenes. Have the students present their scenarios to the whole class.
7. After several sessions working with their characters in various ways, ask students to write (or tell) a brief autobiography of their character.
8. As a culminating activity, have the class write and perform a group play incorporating the characters.

Caveats and Options

1. Videotape any of the classes and review the videotape with the class for the purpose of error correction, community building, or character development.
2. If students begin to tire of the character they created, suggest that they create an alter ego to the character or otherwise change the character. For these activities to be compelling and interesting to students, they have to find their characters interesting to work with.
3. Take on a new character yourself to create an environment in which students will feel it's acceptable to experiment and take risks with their new identities.

References and Further Reading

Boleslavsky, R. (1984). *Acting: The first six lessons.* New York: Theatre Arts Books.

Clark, R. (1987). *Language teaching techniques.* Brattleboro, VT: Pro Lingua Associates.

Polsky, M. (1980). *Let's improvise: Becoming creative, expressive and spontaneous through drama.* Englewood Cliffs, NJ: Prentice Hall.

Spolin, V. (1983). *Improvisation for the theater.* Evanston, IL: Northwestern University Press.

Contributor

Marti Anderson is a faculty member in the Master of Arts in Teaching Program, The School for International Training, Brattleboro, Vermont, in the United States.

The Lover, the Boss, and the Mother

Levels
Any

Aims
Learn how age and social status can affect communication

Class Time
30–45 minutes

Preparation Time
10 minutes

Resources
Script

In this activity, students read the same short two-person scene several times, assuming a different social status each time. The discussion focuses on changes in voice and body language required by different characters and how these changes affect the students' choice of strategies for communication. Students' awareness of differences in tone, intonation, and inflection combined with body language may help them avoid miscommunication in future intercultural settings.

Procedure

1. Divide students into groups of three and explain the activity. While two students are acting, the third member will act as an observer.
2. Give a copy of the script to one member of each group (see the Appendix). Note that one person has the lines and the other must react only.
3. Have two members of each group take turns acting out the same script: first as two lovers, then as a boss and employee, and a third time as mother and child. Have the observer record changes in vocal quality, body language, and personal space.
4. Have the students change roles and repeat Step 3.
5. Focus the postactivity discussion on how the changes in vocal qualities, such as tone, intonation, and inflection, combined with body language and personal space can affect meaning.

Appendix: Sample Script

> Why?
>
> You just don't understand what I've been trying to tell you.
>
> I've tried to tell you again and again.
>
> I just can't take it anymore.

Contributors

Marni Baker and Katharine Isbell developed an intercultural communication workshop that used drama techniques for Japanese students going to study abroad. This activity comes from that workshop.

The Meeting

Levels
Any

Aims
Become aware of how emotions are expressed culturally through body language

Class Time
30-45 minutes

Preparation Time
10 minutes

Resources
Emotion cards

In this activity, students assume and express emotions through their hands, feet, face, and posture while acting out a meeting. Although expressing the same emotions through voice is not the main aim of the activity, students can be given short lines to help them stay in character.

Procedure

1. Ask students to show the three emotions—boredom, aggression, and nervousness—with different parts of their body: hands, face, posture, and finally feet. Students may need prompting and modeling at this point.
2. Divide students into groups of no more than eight students, and put each group at its own table. Ideally, there should be an instructor for each table.
3. Give each group member a card with an emotion written on it. Assume the role of CEO and read an agenda (see the Appendix) while the students act out their parts. As the meeting progresses, have the students express that emotion as if they were attending a real meeting using their hands, face, feet, and posture.
4. Appoint one student at each table an observer who will try to figure out the emotion each member is portraying.
5. Hold new meetings so students have an opportunity to practice each emotion.
6. Focus postactivity discussion on intercultural differences in the expression of emotion and the students' feelings about communicating emotions differently from the way they might in their own culture.

Caveats and Options

1. After students have practiced portraying each emotion through body language, add student-generated lines.
2. Give students a list of short lines and have them deliver any two lines that express the same emotion they are demonstrating through their body language. For example:

> I agree.
>
> That idea make no sense whatsoever.
>
> Whose idea was this?
>
> What do you mean?

Contributors

Marni Baker and Katharine Isbell developed an intercultural communication workshop that used drama techniques for Japanese students going to study abroad. This activity comes from that workshop.

Creative Acts: A Workshop Approach

Levels
Low intermediate;
young adults

Aims
Use mime and
improvisation to create
a two-scene play
Learn how plays can
embody themes relevant
to students' lives

Class Time
2 hours

Preparation Time
None

Resources
One sheet of paper per
student

Procedure

Scene 1

1. Have students sit in a large horseshoe. Explain that they're going to make a 5-minute play in pairs about going on a homestay in the country where they are studying with you right now.
2. Give out one sheet of paper to each student. Ask the students to fold the paper into four parts, and tear or cut out the rectangles.
3. Tell the students to write or draw on each rectangle something that they would pack in their luggage if they were going on a homestay in a foreign country. Ask the class to put their rectangles facedown in the middle of the horseshoe space.
4. Divide the students into groups of four: one actor and three guessers. Have the actor pick up a slip of paper and mime its content to their group. Have the person who guesses right take the next turn as the actor.
5. Ask the students to work in pairs: One person plays a parent; the other, a teenaged daughter or son. They are at home in a foreign country (i.e., not the country where you are right now). Write these questions on the board:
   - Which foreign country do they come from?
   - Why is he or she going on a homestay (holiday, work, language learning)?
   - What is going to be difficult for both the parent and the teenager to get used to?

   Have the pairs discuss and make notes in order to create their roles.

6. Talk your class through the following mime:

    The teenage son or daughter is at home in a foreign country. He or she is packing to go on a homestay for 1 month.

    Son or daughter: Open your suitcase and start packing. When you are ready, close it, lock it, pick it up, and walk downstairs. Give the suitcase to your parent.

    Parent: Stand up and take the suitcase. Open the front door. Go outside and open the trunk of the car. Put the suitcase in. Close the trunk. Lock it.

    Parent and son or daughter: Get in the car and drive to the airport.

7. Brainstorm with the class:
    - typical things a parent says on saying goodbye to their child in such a situation
    - typical things the son or daughter will miss when going abroad for the very first time

    Expand on the students' vocabulary as needed.

8. Rotate pairs, and ask the new pairs to act and speak the scene again, including ideas from Step 7 for the conversation in the car. Ask the pairs to perform getting out of the car at the airport, unloading the suitcase, checking in, and saying goodbye.

9. Ask the pairs to mime getting out of the car at the airport, unloading the suitcase, checking in, and saying goodbye.

10. Finish the first scene by asking the students to write a diary entry in role for their experience of saying goodbye before the homestay starts, with cues such as *What happened today? How did you feel? What is going to happen at the start of the homestay?*

Scene 2

1. As homework preparation, have each pair draw a floor plan of their home in the country where they are studying, labeling important items around the house.
2. In class, divide the students into the same pairs. Have one student take their floor plan and walk the partner through their home, showing interesting details and introducing the family.
3. Have the students act and speak the scene again. Then have them swap roles and repeat both steps.
4. Ask the students to decide which "tour" they want to include in their play. According to their choice, have students choose their roles. The homestay person is the same in both Scenes 1 and 2. The parent in Scene 1 becomes the homestay host in Scene 2.
5. Ask the students to rehearse their play so that it stops in Scene 2 at a point where there is an important misunderstanding between the two characters.
6. Ask each pair to perform their play for another pair.
7. After the performance, ask the students to write a second personal diary entry *in role* about things that were surprising and unexpected at the start of the homestay. Use this entry as a basis for developing the play further, for examining dramatic tension, or for discussing everyday cross-cultural differences.

Caveats and Options

1. After one pair's performance in Step 6, have the spectators ask the actors questions about their homestay experience and assess the individual performance of both actors. Then have the spectator-interviewer use the completed table to give some focused feedback to one of the actors about
   - movement
   - action and gestures
   - loud and clear voice
   - pace
   - storyline

2. The use of diary writing for in-role reflection is an effective way to help students become aware of their own life experiences, attitudes, and values.

References and Further Reading

Scarcella, R. (1978). Socio-drama for social interaction. *TESOL Quarterly, 12*, 41–46.

Wagner, B. J. (1990). *Dorothy Heathcote: Drama as a learning medium*. Cheltenham, England: Stanley Thorne.

Contributor

Andrew Barfield teaches at Tsukuba University, Japan, and enjoys teaching English creatively.

West Side Story: A Lesson

Levels
Beginning;
postsecondary

Aims
Read fictional literature
Learn about style, tone, and voice
Use the text as a reference

Class Time
1 hour

Preparation Time
20 minutes

Resources
Romeo and Juliet/West Side Story (1965)
Audiotape of the music and lyrics

This material was prepared for a reading class at the junior college level.

Procedure

1. Choose a scene or scenes on which to base the lesson.
2. Write an introductory passage to explain the content of the scene(s) to the students before they read it. Include vocabulary and cultural explanations if necessary. (See Appendix.)
3. Assign the scene(s) as reading homework.
4. At the following class session, divide the students into groups of four or five and have them read the scene together, helping each other with vocabulary.
5. Either supply the Spanish vocabulary or (better, if feasible) have Spanish-speaking students explain it to the class.
6. In groups, have students respond to the comprehension questions.
7. As a class or in groups, have students respond to the discussion points, paying special attention to finding support in the text, when appropriate, and offering examples when responding to a more general question or statement.
8. Show the video. Elicit reactions to the performances as well as comments on script differences and on scene sequence. Ask how they affect the reader versus the viewer.
9. Repeat Steps 1-8 for other scenes in the play.

Caveats and Options

1. In a beginning-level class, the level of understanding and enjoyment of the students is directly proportionate to the amount of prereading preparation they receive. This is particularly true for the first scenes of a play. As the students become more familiar and more engaged with

the subject and the characters, cut the amount of preparation back until almost no preparation is necessary for the final scenes.
2. Have the students read for a specific purpose to enhance their understanding and interest. For example, in Act 1, Scene 5 (see the Appendix) ask the students to look for the word *tonight* and think about why it is repeated so frequently. Or ask the students to think about what it is like for an immigrant to live in America or what a real American is before reading the scene.
3. If time permits and if the students enjoy it, engage the students in group singing, which reinforces pronunciation and stress patterns.

References and Further Reading

Shakespeare, W., Laurents, A. (Text), & Sondheim, S. (Lyrics). (1965). *Romeo and Juliet/West Side Story.* New York: Dell.

Appendix: Sample Lesson: Act 1, Scene 5 of *West Side Story*

Introduction to Scene 5

This scene is divided in two parts. In the first part, Tony and Maria are alone together. They talk and sing about their love. The mood is secret and romantic.

In the second part, the Puerto Rican girls and Bernardo talk and sing about being immigrants in America. You will notice that they have mixed feelings: They talk about how immigrants are treated and what is better in America than in Puerto Rico. But Rosalia in particular expresses how homesick immigrants can be for their country.

Puerto Rico has a special relationship with the United States. It is not an American state, but it has special privileges concerning trade and immigration.

Vocabulary
    Spic: an insulting word for Spanish speakers
    Polack: an insulting word for Polish immigrants

Comprehension (*) and Discussion(**) Questions

* What is Maria afraid of at the beginning of the scene?
* Tony says, "I'm *not* one of them." What does he mean?
** Maria says of her father, "He is afraid of you." What does she mean?
** Why is the word *tonight* repeated several times?
* Why does Tony speak Spanish in this conversation?
  Maria: Come to the back door.
  Tony: *Sí*
  Maria: Tony! What does Tony stand for?
  Tony: Anton
  Maria: *Te adoro*, Anton
  Tony: *Te adoro*, Maria
** Who is more realistic, Tony or Maria? Give examples.
* Anita says, "She has a mother. Also a father." What does she mean?
* When Anita yells, "Immigrant!" is it an insult or a compliment?
* Make a list of the good things Rosalia tells about Puerto Rico.
* Make a list of the bad things Anita and the other girls describe about Puerto Rico.
* In this song, what are the advantages of living in America? And the disadvantages?
** Do you think Puerto Rico is beautiful or ugly?
** Think about your position and write your list of what is positive and negative for you in America. Share your list with your group and compare your answers.

** Be an active reader: Think about what you know so far and write down what you predict will happen between:
Tony and Maria
The Jets and the Sharks
Riff and Tony
Bernardo and Maria

After you watch the video: Compare and contrast the text and the video.

* Why were some changes made?

* Which version do you prefer and why?

Contributor

Françoise Beniston developed this material while teaching at Evergreen Valley College, San Jose, California. She is currently the director of a distance learning program in Menlo Park, California, in the United States.

Characters Come to Life

Levels
High beginning +;
secondary +

Aims
Reinforce and expand
understanding of the
characters in a story
Develop speaking and
listening skills

Class Time
30 minutes

Preparation Time
Minimal

Resources
Story, play, or novel
students are currently
reading

Many students enjoy role-playing characters in a story. By having volunteers assume these roles for small-group interviews, students can ask and answer questions using knowledge from readings and their own imaginations.

Procedure

1. List on the board several characters familiar to students from a story, novel, or play they are reading.
2. Ask for volunteers to assume the roles of these characters. They will be interviewed by other students in small groups.
3. Have the role players leave the room and discuss with each other what they know, believe, and imagine about their characters. Have them take their texts with them to consult as needed.
4. With the rest of the students, brainstorm the types of questions they might ask the characters. Write them on the board. Depending on the level of the students, keep the questions on the board or erase them when the role players return.
5. Divide the students into as many small groups as there are characters to interview. Groups of three or four work best. Have each group arrange their chairs or desks in a circle, with an extra seat for the person they will interview.
6. Invite the role players back into the classroom. Have each one join a small group and answer questions from the group members in character. After a few minutes, ask each one to move on to the next group.
7. Follow up with a brief full-class discussion, inviting comments from both role players and interviewers.

Caveats and Options

1. Choose characters about whom the students have sufficient knowledge from the reading to carry out an interview.
2. Welcome invention, but make sure it is linked to the reader's interpretation of the text. The nature of the text will also influence the level of creativity: For example, inventiveness would be more appropriate with a humorous short story than with a novel in which the students are trying to gain insight into the story.
3. When brainstorming questions with the class, review the grammar of question formation. Write the questions on the board as posed by the students and then ask them to edit the questions.
4. Conduct these interviews as a jigsaw activity. Ask all the students to choose a character to play. Have the students who are playing the same character get together to prepare. Then create groups in which each person plays a different character and the students take turns interviewing each other.

Contributor

Linda Butler teaches ESL, writes, and consults in Massachusetts, in the United States. She is the creator of The ESOL Reader's Companion *series (McGraw-Hill).*

Interacting With Literature Via Student-Produced Videos

Levels
High intermediate +

Aims
Develop an interest in literature
Use language skills in a creative video project

Class Time
10 + hours

Preparation Time
Minimal

Resources
Short story or chapter from a novel
Video camera and videotape player

One way to get students excited about literature is to have them produce videos based on what they have read. While they are moving from the page to the camera, students are carefully analyzing the language, plot, and characters of the story as well as exploring different points of view. Most importantly, they are using their language skills to participate in a creative process similar to that of the author whose work they are reading.

Procedure

1. Make sure the students understand the story or novel chapter they will videotape.
2. Help students visualize the written text they will videotape:
   - Take small segments of the text and have the students demonstrate the actions described.
   - Have the students draw pictures depicting different scenes in the story.
   - Have students list adjectives that describe the main characters.
3. Show the students a simple example of the screenplay format. (See the Appendix for an example.)
4. Divide the students into groups to write the first screenplay draft. During the writing process, allow them to change the details of the story if they wish.
5. Collect the screenplays from the groups. Make suggestions for revisions.
6. Have the groups rewrite their screenplays.
7. Allow the students to choose the cast, camera operator, and director for each group. Students with small roles should have additional responsibilities for organizing props or costumes.

8. Rehearse the scenes that will be videotaped. During the rehearsal, the director of each group is in charge and should be making decisions about where the camera will be placed for each scene.
9. Videotape the scenes. If possible, have the director or another group member work the camera; this increases student investment in the project.
10. Show the videos. Try to make an event of it by having awards for each group.

Caveats and Options

1. Choose stories that contain some action or novel passages that demonstrate character development. The selection should be three to five pages long. One short story that works well is Saroyan's (1958) "The Filipino and the Drunkard." Carefully selected scenes from *The Great Gatsby* (Fitzgerald, 1925/1980) and *The Accidental Tourist* (Tyler, 1985) have also been the inspiration for successful student video projects.
2. Encourage students to use the literature selection as a springboard for their videos rather than adapting it word for word. They should add characters, modify the plot, or change the ending of the story if they wish. In this way, they are using their imaginations and becoming more involved in the creative process.
3. Each group will have different interpretations of the story. Therefore, the groups should try to videotape their versions separately. When you show the videotapes to the class, the students will enjoy seeing how the groups interpreted the story.

References and Further Reading

Fitzgerald, F. S. (1980). *The great Gatsby*. New York: Scribner's. (Original work published 1925)

Portnoy, K. (1991). *Screen adaptation, a scriptwriting handbook*. Stoneham, MA: Butterworth-Heinemann.

Saroyan, W. (1958). The Filipino and the drunkard. In *The William Saroyan reader* (pp. 10-12). New York: George Braziller.

Stempleski, S., & Arcario, P. (Eds.). (1993). *Video in second language teaching: Using, selecting, and producing video for the classroom*. Alexandria, VA: TESOL.

Tyler, A. (1985). *The accidental tourist*. New York: Random House.

Appendix: Sample Screenplay Format

- Descriptions of actions begin at the left-hand margin.
- Characters are centered in the middle of the page.
- The dialogue is moved in several spaces from the left and is written under the name of the character who speaks it.
- Descriptions of how the dialogue should be spoken are put in parentheses under the character's name.

The students move around in the chairs, nervously fiddling with their papers, while the teacher, Pamela, is looking at her watch. ← DESCRIPTION OF ACTION

CHARACTER → Pamela

Please take out your homework for today. ← DIALOGUE

The students look around and whisper to each other. ← DESCRIPTION OF ACTION

CHARACTER → Juan

(innocently) ← HOW THE DIALOGUE IS SPOKEN

Homework? What homework? You didn't give us any! ← DIALOGUE

All the students begin to nod their heads vigorously in agreement. ← DESCRIPTION OF ACTION

Contributor

Pamela Couch is an ESL instructor at Boston University, Boston, Massachusetts, in the United States, and supervises the American literature elective classes.

Words in Action

Levels
High beginning

Aims
Practice speaking
Explore the relationship between language and actions in advertising

Class Time
1-2 class hours

Preparation Time
15 minutes

Resources
Videotape player
Videotape of a selection of advertisements from local TV

Caveats and Options

Advertisements grab the attention of the students and act as a stimulus for language production. With this activity students think about the language they need to advertise a product. They see a direct relationship between their actions and the words they use.

Procedure

1. Ask the students to form groups (the same number of groups as the number of advertisements you have).
2. Show the video with no sound.
3. Assign each group one advertisement.
4. Allow the groups 25 minutes to discuss and plan how to act out the advertisement.
5. Tell the students their actions and words have equal importance in the advertisement. Have them decide
   - the language they will use. Provide a variety of resources like dictionaries, newspaper or magazine advertisements, and word lists.
   - the actions they will use. They may choose to use the same actions shown in the video or they can use other actions.
6. Have each group act out its advertisement in English.
7. Show the original again with sound.
8. Have the rest of the class assess the group's performance.

Videotape the students acting out their advertisements.

Contributors

David Gardner is Senior Language Instructor in the English Centre at the University of Hong Kong. Lindsay Miller is Assistant Professor in the English Department at City University of Hong Kong.

Silent Scene

Levels
Any

Aims
Separate action from dialogue
Focus on the action and interpret it verbally

Class Time
15 minutes

Preparation Time
10 minutes

Resources
Role cards

Using a fish bowl approach, students observe two pairs of students working through a scene, one physically, the other verbally.

Procedure

1. Select a collection of writings (e.g., Donovan, Jeffares, & Kennelly's (1994) *Ireland's Women*) from which to choose suitable texts for study.
2. Arrange the seats in a circle, with two chairs in the center.
3. Select four students to perform the scene. Two (A and B) will mime, and the others (a and b) will sit behind A and B on the chairs and speak. Have all other students sit in the circle (see Appendix A).
4. Give A and B each a role card (see Appendix B). Have them read the information on the card and put it away.
5. Have A and B mime the scene while a and b interpret A's and B's action verbally (a speaks for A, and b speaks for B).
6. Have other pairs of students interpret the same scene or other scenes.

Caveats and Options

1. This activity can provide a stimulating introduction to the study of a scene, play, or character, or it can reinforce and check on comprehension of work studied previously.
2. In a subsequent session, compare the improvisation in this activity with the original text.
3. Begin this kind of work with a two-character scene. As students become familiar with the approach, use three- and even four-character scenes.

References and Further Reading

Donovan, K., Jeffares, N., & Kennelly, B. (1994). *Ireland's women*. London: Kyle Cathie.

Appendix A: Seating Plan

```
          X    X  X  X
       X X              X
  X   X  |a|   A     B  |b|        X
      X                    X
         X       X  X  X  X X
```

Appendix B: Role Cards

A	B
* announce your engagement	* announce your engagement to the same person
* show diary proof	* show diary proof
* "He changed his mind."	* "He was entrapped."

Contributor

Geraldine Hetherton is an EFL Lecturer at Fukui Prefectural University, Japan, and has also taught in Europe, Africa, and the Middle East.

Playing With Narratives

Levels
Intermediate +

Aims
Build oral communication and presentation skills
Learn playwriting by converting short narratives into dramatic form

Class Time
4 hours over several sessions

Preparation Time
1 hour

Resources
Copies of a narrative text (e.g., song, story, poem)

In this activity, students use cooperative learning to create bits of dialogue in scenes. In the process they come to understand dramatic and narrative forms, including the elements of the short story, as well as structural features such as beginning, middle, and end; the concept of a scene; and the division of a story into scenes. Through converting narrative to play format, students gain a sense of mastery; build bonds; enjoy an atmosphere of playing that reduces the stress and anxiety of language learning; and practice projecting their voices, speaking clearly, and using appropriate intonation.

Procedure

1. Have the class read and discuss a short piece of narrative for basic comprehension and vocabulary. If it is a song, sing it. Then analyze it in terms of the basic elements of character, structure, setting, theme, plot, and so on.
2. Once the students are familiar with the characters and understand the structure of the story, go through the plot step by step, numbering scenes and describing them in a sentence. (You may want to allow for the creative expansion of the story through additional scenes, such as the one that may have preceded the action.)
3. Assign scenes to groups. Make sure there is a separate scene for each group of two or three students. If the class is large, have two groups work on the same scene.
4. Demonstrate the format for writing dramatic discourse, using an imaginary scene.
5. After the students have had time to put their scenes into written form, collect the scenes. Assist the class in collaboratively compiling the scenes by choosing and editing individual contributions.

6. Distribute copies of the finished product to everyone and do a read-through. Assign parts, rehearse, and have the students perform for each other, either from memory or with script in hand.

Caveats and Options

1. Try to pick a text that affords speaking parts for everyone, whether townspeople, inanimate objects, or a chorus that can be one or more characters. Parts can be shared, and most should be brief.
2. Give all students input into creating and writing their assigned scene. Once the format has been established and the groups have discussed their ideas, they can do some writing at home and some collaboratively in class.
3. If the class is large, and you don't mind a two-ring circus, have different segments of the class work on two different pieces of literature or two parts of the same longer piece. The two segments will still consist of small groups working on their assigned scenes.
4. This activity can be used with all ages and works well with mixed-level groups. For a younger group, "Rudolph the Red-Nosed Reindeer" works very well. For an older group try fairy tales, narrative poems, myths, folktales, or open-ended stories—or to start with something simple, use a popular song that tells a story.

Contributor

Ruth E. Levikoff teaches ESOL in a public school in Philadelphia, Pennsylvania, in the United States. After earning her MA in education, she did graduate study in theater, worked in theater and puppetry, and gave workshops in creative dramatics.

Append a Scene

Levels
Advanced

Aims
Practice writing creatively
Use spoken English communicatively
Read aloud and act
Practice critiquing others' writing

Class Time
2 hours

Preparation Time
None

Resources
Script of a short play in or translated into modern, understandable English

Adding a scene to an existing play enhances students' interest in and understanding of the text as well as their writing skills.

Procedure

1. Have students read the play at home.
2. Discuss the plot and characters with the students in class, clarifying any part in the play that they do not understand.
3. Divide the class into pairs or groups of three.
4. Have each pair or group write a short, original scene that illuminates certain points in- or outside the text: a scene that does not exist in the play, such as a dialogue between two characters discussing an event or a character in the play. Ensure that at least two groups take on the same topic so that the class has a chance to see different points of view at work.
5. Have the pairs or groups playread their scenes, inviting comments from the class on how different pairs or groups treated a given topic, what the strong and weak points in the dialogue were, and how the scene could be improved.

Caveats and Options

1. A good—though not short—play that works well is Ibsen's *A Doll's House* (1879/1992), for which you can have students write a scene between Dr. Rank and Mrs. Linde discussing Nora's character or a scene in which Nora tells Dr. Rank about her secret. (Neither of these scenes exists in the original play.)

2. Have students rewrite the confrontation scene between Nora and Helmer as if they are not Norwegians but rather belonged to the students' nationality or culture.
3. After commenting on the pairs' or groups' work, have them rewrite their scenes.

References and Further Reading

Ibsen, H. (1992). *A doll's house*. New York: Dover. (Original work published 1879)

Contributor

Wisam Mansour is Assistant Professor of English at the Applied Science University, Amman, Jordan.

Playwrite and Learn English

Levels
Advanced

Aims
Practice writing creatively
Use spoken English communicatively
Read aloud and act
Practice critiquing others' writing

Class Time
2 hours

Preparation Time
None

Resources
None

Caveats and Options

By writing a piece of drama together, students can improve their spoken and written English as well as their communication and negotiation skills.

Procedure

1. Split the class into groups of four or five.
2. Ask each group to think of a situation and create a 3- to 5-minute scene with a role for each member in the group. Have a scribe in each group write down the scene.
3. Have each group playread their scene in front of the class.
4. After each performance, have the class point out language and structural errors in the production. Comment as necessary. Have the scribe note your comments on the text.
5. In the next class meeting, have the groups rewrite their vignettes, incorporating in them the remarks made in class.
6. Have the class perform their vignettes again, encouraging further comments from the rest of the class.

With classes larger than 25 students, form groups of 6 or 7 students.

Contributor

Wisam Mansour is Assistant Professor of English at the Applied Science University, Amman, Jordan.

Acting It Out

Levels
High beginning +

Aims
Become sensitive to dialogue
Learn to mime expressively

Class Time
Variable

Preparation Time
Variable

Resources
Realia you want the students to use when they act out the dialogue

When we ask students to act and say their lines at the same time, it's easy for them to get confused. Allowing students to mime a play (or parts of a play) focuses their attention on meaningful motions they will need to use to get the message of the play across.

Procedure

1. Select a play at an appropriate level for the class.
2. Arrange the students into groups. The number in your groups will depend on the number of parts in the play, but additional actors can be used to represent inanimate objects.
3. Divide the reading into sections. Give each group one section.
4. Tell the students that they will have to read through their section and then decide how they can mime the dialogue.
5. Allow the students to find a quiet place (either an empty classroom or a corner of a recreation area). Give them 45 minutes to read their section and decide on how they can mime it.
6. While the students are working on this, circulate and give help in reading the text and suggestions on how to act it out if necessary.
7. Bring the whole class together for the second hour. Have each group act out their section. While one group is acting, the other students in the class can talk out loud about what they think the story is (everyone will have some ideas as they have already read one section of the play).
8. For homework, or in the next lesson, ask the students to read the whole play.

Caveats and Options

1. If you have a long play, you may want to use this idea for only one act/section.
2. Depending on the complexity of the play or the amount of preteaching you have to do, this activity could take place over several lessons.
3. After finishing this task, the students could write a simple play themselves then act it out in front of the class.
4. If your students are not used to acting or miming, it is a good idea to introduce short mime actions in earlier lessons. For example, students can act out one word (occupations, verbs, feelings), phrases, or whole sentences for the other students to guess.
5. The game Charades is a good way to accustom students to the idea of miming to convey a message.

Contributor

Lindsay Miller is Assistant Professor in the English Department at City University of Hong Kong.

Teaching Pronunciation Dramatically

Levels
Low intermediate +;
adolescents or adults

Aims
Improve pronunciation
through guided practice
with stress and rhythm
patterns
Focus on major
sentence stress

Class Time
1 hour initially

Preparation Time
20 minutes

Resources
Two- to five-page
excerpt from a play

Pronunciation specialists emphasize that suprasegmentals play a prominent role in the acquisition of L2 phonology (Morley, 1994; Wong, 1986). This activity uses excerpts from contemporary plays to illustrate the impact of stress, rhythm, and intonation patterns within connected streams of speech.

Procedure

1. Make a sufficient number of copies of a contemporary play excerpt (see Handman, 1978; Schulman & Meckler, 1984).
2. Bring the copies to class and explain to students any necessary background information.
3. Ask students to predict what some characters' problems might be. Write some of these on the board.
4. Read aloud a brief segment from the excerpt, and ask students to write down any individual words, phrases, or sentences they are able to recognize as you talk.
5. Begin a whole-class discussion of the segment they have just heard (e.g., "What did the characters do or say? Did they remind you of any anyone you know?").
6. Distribute copies of the excerpt and ask students to read it through once in silence.
7. Answer students' questions concerning unusual vocabulary or implied meanings. Try to limit the time you spend on this portion of the lesson to no more than 3–5 minutes.
8. Ask students to guess what events might have led up to the events depicted in the excerpt. Alternatively, ask them to predict subsequent events from the play.

9. Initiate the lesson focus on suprasegmentals. Illustrate with a few examples from the excerpt what phonology specialists mean by the term *major sentence stress* (see Caveats and Options). In the following minidialogue, for example, the first time the word *used* is spoken it receives major sentence stress, as does the word *hated* in Speaker A's response:
   A: Did you buy a brand new car last week?
   B: No, I bought a *used* car.
   A: Oh, I thought you *hated* used cars.
10. Caution learners about two important factors: (a) Some sentences may have more than one prominently stressed word (e.g., in cases of comparative stress patterns or longer utterances), and (b) locations of major sentence stress shift subtly depending upon a speaker's intended meaning.
11. Explain that you are not looking for right or wrong answers but simply using the activity as an opportunity to explore ways in which sentence-level stress operates in English. Make clear, however, that patterns of major sentence stress are systematic in English and that there are many identifiable constraints upon their possible locations due to discourse-level meanings.
12. Ask students to read the excerpt again, this time using a pencil to circle any words they believe would receive major sentence stress in the excerpt's individual lines if spoken by a competent actor.
13. After most students have worked through the excerpt, arrange the class in dyads. Have students work with a partner to compare their work and try to reach consensus on as many locations of major sentence stress as time permits.
14. While the partners are trying to reach consensus, encourage them to explain why actors would highlight specific words. Ask them to think about differences in meaning if a speaker were to use major sentence stress in alternative locations.
15. Leave plenty of opportunities for everyone to practice lines from the play aloud in dyads and other class configurations.
16. Throughout these stages, remind students that they do not need to memorize the material. When working with a written script, they

should be exercising their short-term memories only. Their purpose is to become as familiar with the materials as possible in the time available while searching for examples of major sentence stress.
17. Move around the room lending assistance and prompting students as needed. Call students' attentions to particular locations of major sentence stress whenever appropriate.
18. Perform brief sections of the play yourself either with a member of the class or with a colleague.
19. While they are listening to live interpretations, ask students to use their script copies to keep track of possible discrepancies between any major sentence stress locations they have identified and ones they actually hear being used.
20. Periodically, discuss such discrepancies with the whole class.
21. Bring in another segment from the same play (or a different play) and continue the process.
22. Build toward small-group performances of the script, and be sure to leave room for students' extemporaneous interpretations.
23. Intersperse individual group performances with whole-class discussions of major sentence stress locations.
24. Provide opportunities for students to compose their own lines and minidialogues based upon the play's characters.

Caveats and Options

1. This process works best as a recurring activity.
2. The first time you do this activity, a good excerpt to use is from Neil Simon's *The Odd Couple* (Handman, 1978, pp. 232-243).
3. Avery and Ehrlich (1992, p. 75) provide clear illustrations and related discussions. Briefly, any individual sentence of spoken English usually contains one word that receives major sentence stress in comparison with other words within the same sentence or utterance.
4. Use whole sentences from the play to illustrate and provide guided practice with related rhythm patterns and intonation as well. See Prator and Robinett (1985, pp. 58-89) for an inventory and accessible discussion of intonation patterns.
5. Select segments from plays that will be of interest to the group of learners. Look for excerpts featuring lively dialogue and good humor that you surmise can be appreciated by L2 learners.

6. Consult with drama departments at your institution for alternative source materials.
7. Transcripts from segments of contemporary movies are useful too. An advantage is that actual movie segments can be played for students on a videotape player.
8. Be sure to comply with local copyright restrictions when working with published materials.

References and Further Reading

Avery, P., & Ehrlich, S. (1992). *Teaching American English pronunciation*. New York: Oxford University Press.

Handman, W. (Ed.). (1978). *Modern American scenes for student actors*. New York: Bantam Books.

Morley, J. (Ed.). (1994). *Pronunciation pedagogy and theory: New views, new directions*. Alexandria, VA: TESOL.

Murphy, J. (1991). Oral communication in TESOL: Integrating speaking, listening, and pronunciation. *TESOL Quarterly, 25*, 51-75.

Prator, C., & Robinett, B. (1985). *Manual of American English pronunciation* (4th ed.). New York: Holt, Rinehart & Winston.

Schulman, M., & Mekler, E. (1984). *The actor's scenebook*. New York: Bantam Books.

Wong, R. (1986). *Teaching pronunciation: Focus on English rhythm and intonation*. Englewood Cliffs, NJ: Prentice Hall.

Contributor

John M. Murphy is Associate Professor of Applied Linguistics and ESL at Georgia State University. His publications have appeared in the TESOL Quarterly, TESOL Journal, English for Specific Purposes, TESL Canada Journal, Prospect, *and elsewhere.*

Reader's Theater: A Primer on Pronunciation

Levels
Intermediate

Aims
Improve pronunciation

Class Time
Variable

Preparation Time
10 minutes

Resources
Short stories
Poems
Fables

Reader's Theater is the oral presentation of written text. It is much more informal than a class play in that there is no need for students to memorize lines or worry about costumes, sets, cues, props, or casting. It is a classroom activity for any number of students that provides instructed practice in intonation, elision, melody, stress patterns, rhythm, volume, rate, articulation, delivery style, and body language.

Procedure

1. Read the selection to the class.
2. Clarify the meaning of any unfamiliar vocabulary.
3. Go through the selection again line by line, having students repeat each line after you in a choral response.
4. Vary the choral responses. For example,
   - read two lines and have students repeat them in unison
   - gradually increase the size of the chunks to be read (i.e., read two lines, have the students read the next two lines, and so on)
   - alternate lines to be read with students (i.e., read one line, have students read the next)
   - have students practice backward buildup (i.e., have students repeat the last word of a selection in unison, mimicking the teacher, then the last two words, three words, and so on, working backwards)
5. Divide students into small groups or pairs to continue practicing.
6. Depending on the selection, hold the final reading as a choral reading (of a poem, for example) or ask individual students to volunteer to read characters' lines.

Caveats and Options

1. The first three stanzas of *Paul Revere's Ride* (Longfellow, 1861, in Untermeyer, 1942) make an excellent introduction to Reader's Theater for their cultural and literary aspects as well as for the pronunciation practice they afford. The rhythm is definite, and students pick it up easily. You can almost hear the hoofbeats.
2. "The Unicorn in the Garden" (Thurber, 1945/1957) is a classic in U.S. literature that also works well because it puts a new twist on an old story. It has parts for five different characters, but the parts can easily be divided so that every student in the class has lines. For a successful follow-up activity, use the lines as the basis for a strip story.
3. Aesop's "The Tortoise and the Hare" (in Reeves, 1962) is a classic that most students already know. They always seem ready to play with it and enjoy it, perhaps because they don't need to worry about understanding it. The only speaking part is that of the narrator. Divide the number of lines by the number of students present that day, or divide the students into tortoises and hares and have them read in unison, adding gestures (e.g., the determined but sluggish movements of the tortoise and the quick and impetuous motions of the hare).

References and Further Reading

Morley, J. (1991). The pronunciation component in teaching English to speakers of other languages. *TESOL Quarterly, 25*, 481-520.

Reeves, J. (1962). The tortoise and the hare. In *Fables from Aesop retold by James Reeves* (pp. 68-73). New York: Henry Z. Walck.

Thurber, J. (1957). The unicorn in the garden. In *The Thurber carnival* (pp. 168-169). New York: Random House. (Original work published 1945)

Untermeyer, L. (Ed.). (1942). *A treasury of great poems English and American.* New York: Simon & Schuster.

Acknowledgment

We saw Deryn Verity present "The Tortoise and the Hare" at the Harvard Summer School in 1987.

Contributors

Christine Root is the author of several ESL textbooks. She is also a consultant in the field and conducts teacher training workshops. John Dumicich teaches at New York University and Hunter College. He does teacher training for the United States Information Service and is the coauthor of Drawing on Experience *(with Christine Root; McGraw-Hill, 1996).*

Lennie, What Were You Going to Do With All Those Rabbits?

Levels
Intermediate +

Aims
Engage in lively conversation
Check understanding of the assigned literature

Class Time
30–45 minutes

Preparation Time
10 minutes

Resources
Story

Student-generated role plays allow students to gain insight into characters and their motivations. Having created closer connections with the text, students become more invested in their reading and analysis processes.

Procedure

1. For homework, ask students to write three questions that they would like to ask the characters in the story that the class is reading.
2. Collect the questions during the next class.
3. Read through the questions and select eight or nine questions that best lend themselves to interesting discussions.
4. Divide a sheet of paper into as many sections as there are questions. Write one question in each section.
5. Make one copy for every three or four students.
6. Cut up each sheet of questions and paper clip them in packs.
7. Put students in groups of three or four.
8. Give each group one stack of questions, placing them face down in the center of the group.
9. Have the first student draw a card and read the question aloud to the group, making sure that everyone understands it.
10. Have the student who drew the card assume the role of the character being addressed and answer the question.
11. Ask the other students in the group to get the character to give full responses to the question and to disagree with or ask the character to justify the responses.
12. When the group feels that the question has been adequately addressed, have the next student pick a card and begin the process again.

Caveats and Options

1. Encourage the students to push the characters to embellish their responses.
2. Encourage the students to incorporate the characters' personas in their role plays.
3. The questions that the students write often demonstrate what they have and have not understood in a piece of literature.

References and Further Reading

Collie, J., & Slater, S. (1992). *Literature in the language classroom*. Cambridge: Cambridge University Press.

Duff, A., & Maley, A. (1991) *Literature*. Oxford: Oxford University Press.

Contributor

Judy Sharkey teaches at Kansai Gaidai College in Japan. She has also taught in the Middle East, Latin America, and the United States.

Writing a Scene From a Play

Levels
Intermediate +

Aims
Read aloud
Act
Write creatively

Class Time
Variable

Preparation Time
10 minutes

Resources
Scripts of plays

By studying the way that playwrights write their scripts, students can study spoken language. They can act out scenes and try to copy the style by writing their own scenes.

Procedure

1. Have students study a scene from a play.
2. Hand out a scene and discuss it with the class.
3. If possible, play an audiotape of the scene.
4. Divide the students into groups according to the number of roles in the scene.
5. Have students playread the scene a number of times, changing roles.
6. Ask students to predict what comes next in the scene.
7. Have students write the next part of the scene.
8. After you have checked the language, have students act out these scenes.

Caveats and Options

1. Encourage imagination and some overacting.
2. Choose a scene that is not more than two to three pages long.
3. If you have access to a video recorder, film the scenes.
4. Plays that work particularly well are Pinter's (1988) *The Caretaker* and *The Dumb Waiter*.

References and Further Reading

Lazar, G. (1993). *Literature and language teaching.* Cambridge: Cambridge University Press.

Pinter, H. (1988). *The caretaker* and *The dumb waiter.* New York: Grove Weidenfeld.

Contributor

Valerie Whiteson teaches in the graduate English Linguistics program at Bar Ilan University in Israel and is the author of several textbooks.

Part IV: A Mixed Bag

Gunther Schmoliner at Eurocentres, Alexandria, Virginia USA.

Young Playwrights

Levels
Intermediate +

Aims
Practice reading aloud
Act and write creatively

Class Time
Five 45-minute class sessions

Preparation Time
Variable

Resources
Poetry collections and anthologies

In this activity, it is important to explain the poem thoroughly. This will enable the students to write a scene based on the ideas in the poem by using their imaginations and to express their point of view on the poem.

Procedure

1. Explain the poem.
2. Divide the class into groups of four or five.
3. In groups, ask students to brainstorm a scene from the poem that they would like to write and act out. Have the students write out the scene.
4. Have the students act out the scene more than once with students changing roles.
5. Ask students if they can predict what might happen next in the poem and why.
6. After checking the language, ask students to work on the scene at home and write or type them up. (See the Appendix for an example.)
7. Distribute final copies to all students and ask them to add their comments and suggestions.
8. Have students present their comments and suggestions.

Caveats and Options

1. Collect all the students' work in an anthology. Encourage the students to be imaginative.
2. One poem that works particularly well for this activity is "If" (Kipling, 1990).

References and Further Reading

Duff, A., & Maley, A. (1982). *Drama techniques in language learning.* Cambridge: Cambridge University Press.

Hayhoe, J., Taylor, R., & Hayhoe, M. (Eds.). (1991). *Between the lines.* Oxford: Heineman.

Kennelly, B. (Ed.). (1981). *The Penguin book of Irish verse.* London: Penguin Books.

Kipling, R. (1990). *Gunga Din and other favorite poems.* New York: Dover.

Lazar, G. (1993). *Literature and language teaching.* Cambridge: Cambridge University Press.

Scott, D., & Kitchen, D. (Ed.). (1989). *Involved in poetry.* Oxford: Heinemann.

Contributor

Nevine A. Abdel Khalek is Coordinator of the Educational Development and Language Teaching Divisions for the Career Development Center, Cairo, Egypt.

Jumpstart Discussion With Think/Pair/Share

Levels
Any

Aims
Increase engagement and participation in class
Rehearse before volunteering in class discussions

Class Time
A few minutes

Preparation Time
None

Resources
Story, novel, or play
Pen and paper (optional)

Think/Pair/Share is an easy-to-use and versatile cooperative learning technique. It involves all members of the class in discussion by getting them thinking, writing, and talking to partners and makes the following full-class discussion livelier and richer.

Procedure

1. Pose a challenging question to the entire class based on the story, novel, or play they are reading or one that is related to some reading they are about to do. The best questions for this activity have more than one possible answer.
2. Give students up to a minute to think about how they would answer the question. If you want students to write down their thoughts, give them more time.
3. Have the students turn to a partner to share their ideas.
4. Call the whole class back together, and ask for volunteers to share their answers with the class.

Caveats and Options

1. You can use this technique at any point during a class discussion, not just to get it started.
2. The question posed to the class can be one that has been raised by a student.
3. Silence in your classroom may feel uncomfortable at first, but don't cut short the time given for thinking.
4. When students write down their thoughts, there is a better chance that the shy ones will also voice their ideas.

5. If you ask students to write their responses, collect them afterwards (to see what they think and be sure they have used the time well). However, be sure students see this writing as a thinking tool, not as producing something to satisfy the teacher.
6. Rather than following the talking in pairs with a full-class discussion, have each set of partners join another pair. (There is value in having students think about an issue and articulate their thoughts even if they are not validated by the instructor in front of the whole class.) Ask the four students to point out similarities and differences in their ideas.
7. If the students are already organized into ongoing small groups or learning teams, ask that they pair off with someone from their group and then join the others in the group to share what they have discussed before going on to further group discussion or other tasks.

References and Further Reading

Johnson, D. W., Johnson, R. T., & Smith, K. A. (1991). *Cooperative learning: Increasing college faculty instructional productivity* (ASHE-ERIC Higher Education Report No. 4). Washington, DC: The George Washington University.

Lyman, F. (1989, September/October). Rechoreographing: The middle-level minuet. *The Early Adolescence Magazine,* pp. 22-24.

Millis, B. J., & Cottell, Jr., P. G. (1995). A cooperative learning structure for large classes: Think-pair-share. *Cooperative Learning and College Teaching, 5,* 13-15.

Contributor

Linda Butler teaches ESL, writes, and consults in Massachusetts, in the United States. She is the creator of The ESOL Reader's Companion *series (McGraw-Hill).*

When a Pig Builds a Bungalow: Working With Titles

Levels
Low intermediate +

Aims
Talk about a story
Become more aware of syntactic patterns and word forms

Class Time
1 hour

Preparation Time
30 minutes

Resources
Story the class has read recently
Short handouts (optional)

In this activity students create a new title for a story they have read. It gives them a chance to talk about the meaning of the story while increasing their awareness of titles as necessary and full-fledged parts of writing and as grammatical entities that are different from the sentence. Students focus on syntax and morphology by playing with words in small, interesting segments. The activity also provides a review of the parts of speech; seems to cut down on the number of students who confuse titles with topic sentences, and titles with thesis statements; and decreases the occurrence of a small but persistent error, ending titles with periods.

Procedure

1. After discussing the story, including the plot, characters, and theme, ask the students about the title: Is it a "grabber" that attracts their attention? Why or why not? Do they like it? What is the purpose of a title? Is this one suitable?
2. Ask them if a title is a sentence. When they answer that it is usually not, tell them that's why the title doesn't end with a period. Tell them it's usually a word or phrase. (Point out that the main words of a title—first, last, and everything in between except articles and prepositions—are capitalized.)
3. Ask the students to think of titles of stories, books, or movies that they like. As they begin to come up with examples, write them on the board. Ask: "Is this a good title? Why? Is it based on the plot, a character, or the theme? Is it a word, a phrase, or (rarely) a sentence?" Ask what part of speech each word in the title is and label the words (see Appendix A). Try to elicit a list of 10 titles.

4. Tell the students to pretend that a movie is going to be made from the story that they have just read and that the producers want to change the title to one that will really make people want to see it. In groups of three or four, have students each choose one of the titles on the board and, using its exact syntactic pattern, create a new title (see Appendix B). Base the title on the plot of the story or a main character or the theme.
5. After 10 minutes, have each group choose one best title to present to the class, explaining why they think it's good. Encourage the students to pitch their titles as a salesperson would. Put the four or five titles on the board, and have the class vote on the one they like best.

Caveats and Options

1. Ask for good titles in the students' L1s that they can translate into English.
2. When the students break into groups, give each student a title to work with that is different from that of everyone else in the group. But allow them to help each other; that's the purpose of putting them in groups.
3. Before you have students make new titles, be sure they have seen several examples analyzed according to parts of speech.
4. Make sure the students change every main word in the title unless it's really impossible.
5. Have the students make posters advertising their movies. Bring in construction paper, markers, crayons, magazines to cut pictures from, scissors, and glue. The more materials you make available, the more creative the students will be.

Appendix A: Parts of Speech, Definitions, and Examples

noun—name of person, place, or thing
    pig, house, wolf, stick, bricks, Porky Pig, Mr. Willard Wolf
pronoun—substitute for a noun
    I, you, she, it, him, her, they, them, my, mine, our, ours
verb—tells what somebody or something *does* or *is*
    built, has eaten, has been eaten, is, was, seemed
adjective—describes (modifies) a noun
    little pig, *cunning* wolf, *flimsy* house, *hefty* appetite, *big* problem

adverb—modifies a verb (often tells how, how often, when)
    quickly, carelessly, lazily, usually, already, yet
preposition—little word with noun or pronoun object
    in the house, *on* the roof, *behind* the pig, *about* three pigs
conjunction—connects words, phrases, clauses, or sentences
    and, but, because, while, although
article—makes a noun specific or nonspecific
    a, an, the
interjection—sudden, short utterance usually expressing emotion
    Ugh! Yikes! Uh-oh!

Appendix B: Creating New Titles

Students copy the titles on the board into the first column. They write the grammatical analysis in the second column and their new titles in the third column.

Sample Title	**Analysis**	**New Title**
The	article	*The*
Most Dangerous	adjective (superlative)	*Most Prudent*
Game	noun	*Pig*
Ghost	noun	*Wolf*
Fried Green	2 adjectives	*Barbecued Pork*
Tomatoes	plural noun	*Chops*
at	preposition	*at*
the	article	*the*
Whistlestop Cafe	2 nouns	*Stick Restaurant*

Contributor

Lynne Davis is an Instructor at the Center for English as a Second Language, Southern Illinois University, Carbondale, Illinois, in the United States.

Put a Ring Around the Thing

Levels
Intermediate +

Aims
Become involved in a literary selection
Share imagined pictures
Expand vocabulary
Engage in conversation

Class Time
15-25 minutes

Preparation Time
5-10 minutes

Resources
Literary selection
Photocopies of a description from the selection

Almost all literary selections, whether short stories, poems, novels, or plays, include within their content or theme an object that proves significant to the advancement of plot or theme. This activity uses such an object as a prereading ploy that arouses students' curiosity and creates interest in the selection to be studied.

Procedure

Before Class

1. Find a description of the object you wish to use in your reading selection. It need not be an exact description, simply a paragraph where the object is first mentioned in the selection. An example is the following description of a hat from O'Connor's (1969) "Everything That Rises Must Converge."

    It was a hideous hat. A purple velvet flap came down on one side of it and stood up on the other; the rest of it was green and looked like a cushion with the stuffing out. He decided it was less comical than jaunty and pathetic. Everything that gave her pleasure was small and depressed him. (p. 32)

2. Make as many copies as you have students in your class.

In Class

1. Ask students to name parts or components of the object you have in mind. For the example above, ask: "What can one use to make a hat?"
2. Appoint a student secretary to write up responses on the board. For the example above, you might get *velvet, feathers, felt, beads, flowers,* or *buttons.*

3. Play some soft background music and ask students to close their eyes and visualize the object chosen. Ask them to see its color and size and to imagine it from several angles. Ask them to imagine it in a shop window. Then ask them to imagine a person walking up to the object and using it. For the example above, ask students to visualize a person going up to a mirror and putting on the imagined hat.
4. Have students stand and mingle, describing their imagined objects to each other.
5. Tell students a few basic facts about the selection you are about to read (for O'Connor's story, tell them that this is a story about a mother and her grown son in a small U.S. town in the 1960s). Tell them that the object they have imagined contributes to the plot or theme of the selection.
6. Ask the students to predict how the object might be important in the selection.
7. Hand out the description of the object. Read the description several times with your students, and have them guess details not clearly revealed. For example, in the O'Connor selection, ask, "Who are the people? What is the relationship between them? How do they feel about each other? Why do you think that they have these feelings?"
8. Ask students if they want to add to their initial predictions.
9. Begin reading the selection and ask students to look for the appearance of the object.
10. As you proceed through the reading of the selection, make students aware of how their attitudes toward the object might change and develop.

Caveats and Options

1. In a large and boisterous class, substitute the mingling stage in Step 4 with pair work in seats.
2. Artistically inclined students may enjoy drawing the object.
3. I have used this activity successfully with Shelley's "Ozymandias" (in 1945 edition), in which the object was an ancient object; Joyce's (1932/1993) "Eveline," in which the object was a picture of a priest; O. Henry's (1909/1969) "The Retrieved Reformation," (The story of Jimmy Valentine) where the object was a toolbox; and Tyler's (1986) *The Accidental Tourist*, where the object was a suitcase.

References and Further Reading

Collie, J., & Slater, S. (1991). *Literature in the language classroom*. Cambridge: Cambridge University Press.

Henry, O. (1969). A retrieved reformation. In *Tales of O. Henry* (pp. 201-204). Garden City, NY: Doubleday. (Original work published in 1909)

Joyce, J. (1993). Eveline. In *The Dubliners* (pp. 29-35). London: Sinclair-Stevenson. (Original work published 1932)

O'Connor, F. (1969). Everything that rises must converge. In *3 by Flannery O'Connor* (pp. 30-35). New York: Signet Classics.

Shelley, P. B. (1945). Ozymandias. In *The best of Shelley* (p. 96). New York: Ronald Press.

Tyler, A. (1986). *The accidental tourist*. New York: Berkeley.

Contributor

Natalie Hess is the author of textbooks for students and teachers. She has taught students and teachers in several countries.

Walk For a Good Talk

Levels
Intermediate +

Class Time
45 minutes

Preparation Time
5-10 minutes

Resources
Story, poem, or novel that the class has read

Teachers enjoy a good discussion in their classrooms, and most students have opinions about stories, poems, novels or plays that they have read. The classroom, however, can often become distancing territory—the place where the right answer is more important than what students think about a problem or how they feel about an issue. This task-based discussion activity makes the task seem nonthreatening and serves as a mask for a genuine opinion exchange.

Procedure

Before Class

1. Write a list of 10 thought-provoking statements that relate to a story, poem, play, or novel that you have just finished reading.
2. Make five or six copies of this list and post them in various places on the walls of your classroom. For "Snow White and the Seven Dwarves," the list might be as follows:
   - Snow White is disgustingly submissive.
   - The true heroine of this story is obviously the queen. At least she tries to change her destiny.
   - The voice in the mirror is the dangerous voice in this story.
   - Snow White is pure and blameless femininity. This is why the story has been loved for so many years.
   - The dwarves are outcasts in society. This is why Snow White loves them. She is an outcast too.
   - The hunter is the real hero of the story.
   - Snow White is a great role model for little girls.

- The only way Snow White can be brought back to life is with a kiss from a man. What a terrible lesson for little girls!
- Her role as housekeeper for little men is the kind of servitude women should be afraid of.
- I don't believe that Snow White will be happy with her prince.

In Class

1. Hand each student an index card and a paper clip.
2. Tell the students that the lists of statements posted about the room are all the same. Have the students go to any list, choose two statements that they agree with and one statement that they disagree with, write the numbers (not the text) on the index card, and pin the card on themselves. As students cluster around the lists reading them, circulate and explain vocabulary.
3. When most students have chosen their numbers, have them walk about the room, find a person that agrees with them on at least one item, and explain to each other why they agree. Give this phase plenty of time (15-20 minutes).
4. Have the students find someone who disagrees with them on one of the items and convince the person who disagrees with them of the rightness of their position. Because by now students will have forgotten what the numbers stand for, have them reread the list together with their new partner (10-15 minutes).
5. Have the students approach the lists and pick a statement that they in some way find interesting but had to omit the previous time because they were allowed to choose only three statements.
6. In small groups, have the students read the statement to each other and explain why they found the statement interesting.
7. As a class, have the students explain why they changed or did not change their opinion about something. Encourage questions and comments.

Caveats and Options

1. The activity will work best if you outline the process and have one or two students repeat the instructions before the first step of the activity.
2. Don't worry if students return to the list many times to read and reread the statements. This only creates greater clarity and brings about more interesting discussion.
3. In Step 2 students will invariably complain that two statements for agreement and one for disagreement are not enough. This makes Step 5 doubly welcome.

References and Further Reading

Bassnett, S., & Grundy, P. (1993). *Language through literature.* Burnt Mill, England: Longman.

Duff, A., & Maley, A. (1990). *Literature.* Oxford: Oxford University Press.

Hess, N. (1991). *Head starts.* Burnt Mill, England: Longman.

Ur, P. (1981). *Discussions that work.* Cambridge: Cambridge University Press.

Contributor

Natalie Hess is the author of textbooks for students and teachers. She has taught students and teachers in several countries.

Choral Chant

Having students create their own chants is a more enjoyable way to check their understanding of character and plot than asking them straightforward comprehension questions. This lively activity also reinforces and follows up on class and individual study of a tale.

Levels
Any

Aims
Understand a story better by transposing it into a simpler form

Class Time
30 minutes

Preparation Time
5 minutes

Resources
Story (written or oral)
Worksheet
Overhead projector (optional)

Procedure

1. Read or tell the story under study, or have students read it silently in class or as a homework assignment.
2. Distribute the worksheet (see Appendix A) and have the students individually, in pairs, or in small groups fill in the chart, noting characters, their main actions, and what they say or a sound that could represent them.
3. Set a pattern or rhythm. Display it on a board or overhead projector. Explain to the students that they must fit the information they have noted on the chart into that pattern. Demonstrate if necessary by writing the first verse with the whole class (see Appendix B).
4. In pairs or groups, have the students write their verses according to the set pattern.
5. Have the students perform their compositions.

Caveats and Options

1. Folktales, fairy tales, and short stories are very suitable for this activity.
2. If you divide the story into sections and assign a section to each group, the class will be able to perform a more interesting choral chain than if everyone works on the whole story. More detail and subtlety can thus be incorporated.
3. Assign roles to groups of students (e.g., narrator, Character A, Character B). Pool the verses and have the groups perform their roles in choral chant.

4. Subdivide each group that has been assigned a role into Speakers and Sound Effects. Have the Speakers chant the dialogue while the Sound Effects maintain a continuous chant in the background (see Appendix B).

References and Further Reading

Carroll, L. (1865). *Alice's adventures in wonderland.* London: Macmillan.

Appendix A: Sample Worksheet

CHARACTER	ACTION	SOUND

Appendix B: Sample Chant

Story: *Alice in Wonderland* (Carroll, 1865)
Roles: Alice (A)
      White Rabbit (W)
      Narrator (N)
  A. A "I'm sleepy," N said Alice, A "I'm sleepy."
     W "I'm late," N said White Rabbit, W "I'm late."
     A "I'm sleepy." N "I'm late."
     A "I'm sleepy." N "I'm late."
     A+N "Oh dear, oh dear, oh dear."
  B. Chanters: accompanying Alice: "Aw-awh" (yawn)
               accompanying White Rabbit: "Tick-tock"

Contributor

Geraldine Hetherton is an EFL Lecturer at Fukui Prefectural University, Japan, and has also taught in Europe, Africa, and the Middle East.

Words They Can Keep

Levels
Intermediate +

Aims
Learn vocabulary in depth

Class Time
2-5 hours

Preparation Time
1 hour

Resources
Literature text
Activity worksheets
Dictionaries

Students need to learn vocabulary words they can make their own—that is, speak with, think with, and solve both personal and academic problems with. Teachers can promote acquisition in depth by encouraging students to interact with the words (a) in a communicative setting and (b) through activities that engage them on both the conceptual and the affective levels, which Vygotsky (1994) and others believe to be closely interrelated. The study of literature provides the perfect setting for these types of activities.

Procedure

1. From the literature text you are using, make up three activity sheets. Sheet A asks students to identify which characters are described by certain target words, Sheet B poses problems for which the solution depends on understanding other words, and Sheet C calls for personal responses using a third set of words. (See the Appendix.)
2. Assign each activity sheet first as homework to be done individually.
3. Assign the first two sheets as group work. (This will probably take more than one class period.) Using the text and the dictionary as resources, have students discuss each question until they reach a reasonable agreement. At this point, ask one student to write down the group's answer, which includes evidence from the text and reference to a page number.
4. Read responses to Sheet C aloud with permission from the writer.

Caveats and Options

1. Groups of three or four work best. Be available to clarify word meanings if a group really seems to be stuck.
2. The target vocabulary can be either words from the text that have already been discussed in class or new words. The second option

presents the additional challenge of trying to apply the dictionary definition of an unfamiliar word to a literary character or situation. Though this tends to be frustrating, it often leads to intense discussions and can also serve to bring home the limitations of dictionary definitions.
3. Give lower level (or underprepared) groups help in locating answers. Depending on need, this help can take the form of chapter, act, scene, or even page numbers. Students still have to come up with explanations for their answers.
4. Students will be more involved with the activities if they are interested in the characters and situations they are reading about. Make sure the text is personally relevant and motivating.

References and Further Reading

Brumfit, C. (1984). The Bangalore procedural syllabus. *ELT Journal, 34,* 233-241.

Carter, R., & Long, M. (1987). *The web of words: Exploring literature through language.* Cambridge: Cambridge University Press.

Ellis, R., Tanaka, Y., & Yamazaki, A. (1994). Classroom interaction, comprehension, and the acquisition of L2 word meanings. *Language Learning, 44,* 449-491.

Leaf, J. (1993). *Creating conversational contexts for reading vocabulary.* Presentation at PennTESOL East Conference, Ursinus College, Collegeville, PA.

Shakespeare, W., & Laurents, A. (Text), Sondheim, S. (Lyrics). (1965). *Romeo and Juliet/West Side Story.* New York: Dell.

Vygotsky, L. (1994). Imagination and creativity of the adolescent. In R. Van der Veer & J. Valsiner (Eds.), *The Vygotsky reader* (pp. 266-288). Oxford: Blackwell.

Appendix

Sample Selections From Activity Sheets Based on *West Side Story*

Though scene numbers are included for the first sheet, some questions could have more than one answer.

A. Specific questions about characters:
   1. Who has a *premonition*? (I, ii)
   2. Who expresses *solidarity*? (I, ii)
   3. Who does something *clandestinely*? (I, v)
   4. Who is *exhilarated*? (I, v)
   5. Who *manipulates* someone? (I, ii)

B. More general problems:
   1. Who is more *chauvinistic*, Riff or Bernardo?
   2. Why does Anita *resent* Tony?
   3. Why do you think the gang members look *detached* at the dance?

C. Personal response questions:
   1. Name someone who is *bespectacled*.
   2. What are you *awed* by?
   3. What is something you have *fancied*?
   4. What are you *nostalgic* about?
   5. What *disguise* would you like to wear to a costume party?

Contributor

Claudia Gellert Schulte teaches high school ESOL in Philadelphia, Pennsylvania, in the United States. She holds an MA in TESOL from Temple University and is currently working on her doctorate there.

Connections

Levels
Intermediate +

Aims
Learn to think and communicate
Acquire vocabulary
Examine style, mood, and theme through word grouping

Class Time
1–2 hours

Preparation Time
Little or none

Resources
Literary texts

Group work in which students sort words into general categories can encourage conceptual thinking and promote communication. It may also promote vocabulary acquisition as a result of (a) interacting closely with the words, (b) communicating and negotiating with partners, and (c) forming associative networks in the mind—as long as these call for loose associations between various types of words as opposed to the close similarities that have been found to interfere with learning. Sorting can also lead to new ways of understanding a literary text and even provide a basis for observations about style, mood, and theme.

Procedure

1. As you read through the text with your students, keep a list of all new or unfamiliar words that are identified and discussed (there should be at least 100). Distribute the list.
2. In groups of three or four, have students sort words into categories suggested by the types of words found on the list. (See Caveats and Options.)
3. Read each group's results aloud to the class.
4. Discuss with the class what the various groupings of words reveal about the style, mood, and theme(s) of the work in question. (See the examples in the Appendix.)

Caveats and Options

1. Depending on the students' level, experience, preparedness, and other factors, (a) set the categories yourself, (b) arrive at the categories through whole-class discussion, or (c) have individual groups choose the categories.
2. Once the categories are chosen, have students assign words to them by either completing one category at a time or going down the

master list and deciding which one each word belongs in. Both approaches are probably equally good; groups should make the choice.
3. Some groupings of words may lend themselves to forming subcategories. You may want to present this as a further option and give examples (see the Appendix).
4. In the master list, include idioms, expressions, and slang words in addition to standard words.
5. A vocabulary approach can only cover some aspects of style, mood, and theme. It is not intended as a means for conducting a comprehensive literary analysis.

References and Further Reading

Nation, I. S. P. (1990). *Teaching and learning vocabulary.* Boston: Heinle & Heinle.

Shakespeare, W., Laurents, A. (Text), & Sondheim, S. (Lyrics). (1965). *Romeo and Juliet/West Side Story.* New York: Dell.

Appendix

Sample Categories From *West Side Story* and Possible Implications for Style, Mood, and Theme

A. Strong action words: *clobber, slither, flail, huddle, hurl, shove, round out, jockey, whirl, zoom, jazz it, rock it, mambo, cha-cha, reel, rumble, lick, jump, lunge, trip up, run him through, dueling, get crackin', gassin', crabbin', twitchin', cannonballin', free-for-all.*
   Style: Dialogue contains many slang words and expressions.
   Mood: Strong physical action, much of it sudden, violent, fast-paced. Overall feeling of restlessness.

B. Words for emotional states: *frenetic, ruefully, anguished, panicky, bravado, chaotic, neurosis, detached, tension, hostility, horrified, triumphant, exultant, glee, festive, fizzy, sunny.*
   Mood: Hopefulness and exhilaration against a pervasive background of restlessness and negativity.

C. Words with negative and positive connotations: *Whacky, venom, stool pigeon, hoodlum, scrawny, pathetic, creep, burlesque, musty, quaint, savagely, yellow-bellied chicken, sardonic, broads, depraved, schmuck, juvenile delinquent, pretty boy, social disease, madwoman, spicks, micks, wop, crazy boy, pig, tramp, garlic mouth, village idiot. Glee, stunning, entrancing, nostalgic, triumphant, exultant, break through.*
(Subcategories: derogatory "names" in general; ethnic slurs as a further subcategory)

    Mood: Mainly negativity, hostility and conflict; some joy and optimism

    Themes: Intolerance and bigotry; their negative effects on all concerned.

Contributor

Claudia Gellert Schulte teaches high school ESOL in Philadelphia, Pennsylvania, in the United States. She holds an MA in TESOL from Temple University and is currently working on her doctorate there.

Thinking Through Metaphors

Levels
Intermediate +

Aims
Understand how metaphors work
Practice conversation in small groups

Class Time
45-60 minutes of one class
15 minutes + of a subsequent class

Preparation Time
10 minutes

Resources
Short poem containing a metaphor or metaphors

The idea of the integrated activities here is to begin with the metaphor as literary language in a poem, to move toward ordinary language by asking students to make metaphors themselves in small-group discussion, and (in a subsequent class) to discuss instances of metaphorical language the students have collected from everyday reading and speech.

Procedure

Activity 1

1. Avoiding metalanguage as much as possible, briefly explain that a metaphor is a word or an expression that defines one thing in terms of another, as in *she is a jewel*. Metaphorical language like this is not literally true but invites us to understand what is said by analyzing the comparisons involved. All metaphorical expressions may ultimately be reduced to formulas of the sort *X is Y*. In the sentence *The rabbit shot through the gate*, for example, the verb is metaphorical, but we analyze this by understanding that *the rabbit* is being compared to or defined as a projectile or bullet.
2. Have students study a short poem that contains some metaphorical language. (See References and Further Reading.)
3. Hand out the poem, clarify any especially difficult vocabulary items, ask the students to find the metaphors, and call attention (if need be) to the particular metaphor or metaphors the implications of which they will go on to explore.
4. Divide the students into pairs or small groups of no more than four.
5. Ask students to focus on the metaphors and list the qualities of the objects named that make the metaphor meaningful. (If *she is a jewel* is in the poem, for example, have students list such qualities of jewels

as *rarity, preciousness, brightness*, and *clarity*. Not all qualities may be relevant in context: *smallness* and *hardness*, for example.)
6. Have students rank these qualities in terms of their relevance in their context, which is the poem.
7. Ask students in their groups to formulate a statement about the central meaning of the poem.
8. Compare and discuss these various formulations with the class as a whole.

Activity 2

1. In their groups, have students make metaphors themselves. Provide the nominal subject, such as *our school*, or perhaps *love*.
2. After students have come up with half a dozen metaphors or more, ask students to rank the metaphors in terms of their plausibility or meaningfulness.
3. Ask the groups to share their findings with the class as a whole and explain their ranking. As in the previous discussion of the poem, this explanation of the ranking will involve an analysis of qualities that seem relevant in context: For example, "In what ways is our school like a temple? And in what ways not?"

Activity 3

1. For a subsequent class, ask students to collect on their own examples of metaphors in everyday speech and from their reading in English. Explain that this is going to be a friendly competition to see who can come up with the most metaphors.
2. In class, ask individual students to read out their lists. Have any other students with the same metaphor raise their hands. Do not count metaphors held in common. Declare the person with the most metaphors left at the end the winner.
3. In summing up, point out metaphors related to ones that students have been airing. Often the metaphorical links come quickly and spontaneously. Once one starts to think in terms of argument as a kind of warfare, for example, one may be reminded of a host of

metaphorical expressions: we *undermine opponents;* adopt *strategies* in order to *shoot down* the arguments of others; *attack* and *defend positions;* and *win* or *lose.*

4. Call attention to any metaphors mentioned by the students that seem especially interesting or expressive of the culture from which they have come. Metaphors may range from the most trivial of expressions—*small potatoes*—to the most profound.

Caveats and Options

1. Some good poems for this activity are "A Poison Tree," by William Blake; "The Eagle," by Alfred Lord Tennyson; "I like to see it lap the miles," by Emily Dickinson; "Nothing Gold Can Stay" or "Fire and Ice," by Robert Frost; and "Morning Song" and "Mirror," by Sylvia Plath. (See the Appendix for a poem that works well, with specific examples of questions and suggestions.)
2. To shorten the time spent on the second activity, offer your own lists. If the nominal subject is, for example, *our school*, a list of metaphors might be *a prison; a tomb; a temple; a museum; a maze; a beehive; a factory; a market; a boat for luxury cruises.* From this list, have the students follow the analytical procedures outlined for Activity 2. The question underlying the discussion towards which the students will be moving is: *What sense does it make to think of your school in any of these terms?*
3. For elaboration of the third activity, draw on Lakoff and Johnson (1980), who have analyzed many instances of metaphor in everyday language to help develop student insights.

References and Further Reading

Carter, R., & Long, M. L. (1987). *The web of words.* Cambridge: Cambridge University Press. (See especially chapter 6, "Words and Their Impact")

Cox, H., & Latham, E. C. (Eds.). (1977). *Selected prose of Robert Frost.* New York: Holt, Rinehart & Winston.

Ellmann, R. (Ed.). (1976). *The new Oxford book of American verse.* New York: Oxford University Press.

Gray, R. (Ed.). (1973). *American verse of the nineteenth century.* London: J. M. Dent & Sons.

Hughes, T. (Ed.). (1981). *The collected poems of Sylvia Plath.* New York: Harper & Row.

Lakoff, G., & Johnson, M. (1980). *Metaphors we live by.* Chicago: University of Chicago Press.

Marsh, G. (1988). *Teaching through poetry.* London: Hodder & Stoughton. (See especially chapter 4, "Mucking About in Words")

Untermeyer, L. (Ed.). (1942). *A treasury of great poems English and American.* New York: Simon & Schuster.

Wordsworth, W. (1975). She dwelt among the untrodden ways. In T. Hutchinson & E. de Selincourt (Eds.), *The poetical works of William Wordsworth* (p. 86). New York: Oxford University Press. (Original work published 1799)

Appendix: Sample Exercise

The following questions might accompany the poem "She dwelt among the untrodden ways" by William Wordsworth (1799/1975).

1. Have students pick out or draw their attention to the metaphors in the middle stanza, which compare Lucy first to a violet, then to a star.
2. In pairs or small groups, have the students list the qualities of the flower and of the star that may be relevant to a comparison with the young woman. (The students may need a little guidance, where the flower is concerned, as violets may be unknown to them. That a violet has a small blossom and grows in shade are perfectly relevant to the ideas and feelings the poet is conveying.)
3. Have students list the qualities of the mossy stone and the black night sky that stand in contrast to the flower and star.
4. Then have students in their pairs or groups formulate a statement about the main meaning of the poem. What is the poet saying about this young woman and her relation to her surroundings? How, in other words, do these metaphors of the flower and star help characterize her, define her relation to the world around her, and suggest the poet's feelings about her? Could the apparently stolid, massively indifferent world around her be in some sense necessary to the appreciation of her qualities?

Contributor

Hardy C. Wilcoxon is a member of the English Department at the Chinese University of Hong Kong, where he teaches literature and coordinates a writing program.